Keep positive!

Lauren Bogat

Be a GREAT FRIEND

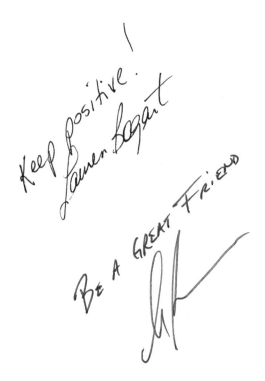

Find your chapter!

Amy Smith

Knowing Pains

Women on Love, Sex and Work in Our 40s

**Old Enough to Know Better,
Young Enough to Do Something About It**

Edited by
Molly Tracy Rosen

WingSpan Press

Printed in the United States of America

Published by WingSpan Press, Livermore, CA
www.wingspanpress.com

The WingSpan name, logo and colophon are the trademarks of
WingSpan Publishing.

ISBN 978-1-59594-254-8

First edition 2009

Library of Congress Control Number 2008933933

Book design by Laura Batti
Cover photography by Holly Stewart

To my mother, the first 40-something woman I ever knew,
who taught me the importance of female connection.
You are still my model of kindness, leadership and grace.
I miss you.

To Team Rosen
Seth, Caleb and Ellie – my lifelong loves and
the best supporters I could ever hope for.

To the honest, inspiring group of women
who brought a fledgling idea to life.

Table of Contents

Introduction

Knowing Pains: Women on Love, Sex and Work in Our 40s is a series of personal essays by successful women from a variety of backgrounds in education, business, and the arts. The growing pains of youth that caused our legs to ache in the middle of the night are over. They left us stronger, bigger and grown up. The "knowing pains" of mid-life are also painful, and also sometimes wake us in the night. They are caused by experiences that are hurtful at the time, but leave us wiser, more empathetic and oftentimes more confident and resilient to take on the experiences that lie ahead. They may be sudden – caused by the death of a parent, by the desertion of a spouse, or by a career failure. They may be gradual and internal – as we understand and accept our strengths and shortcomings. Knowing pains may be caused by positive experiences too, like rediscovering our passions and letting ourselves fully enjoy pleasures like our favorite musician, yoga or hiking with a close friend.

Throughout our lives, we've played different roles such as daughter, student or friend. We have even had different shoes for our different activities such as going to school or church. Yet at this stage in our lives, we have more roles to play than ever before, as professional, friend, wife, volunteer, mother. These roles are reflected in the pile of assorted shoes amassed in our closet or by the front door. Work pumps, casual flats, strappy sandals, running shoes, flip-flops. Instead of hats representing our various roles, it's now shoes. The illustrations in this book reflect the variety of roles and the variety of voices represented in the stories ahead.

You will meet Natalie who reports on her "hair experiment," and Ona who tries a different kind of experiment through a love triangle. Get inspired by the passions of Nancy and Ana. Share the heartache of Maria and Regina. Samantha, a software project manager, shares her experience of being single and dating at 40. Lori, a nonprofit consultant, shares the humor of being a "geriatric mama." Elizabeth talks about her acceptance of God. Elaine talks about her rejection of retail store dressing rooms.

These women are the women around you – the women in your life who have a story to tell. These are the women in our lives who get more interesting, more kind, and more powerful as they navigate rocky relationships, social expectations and their own dreams. Some are married. Many are not. Some have children. Others do not.

Never would I identify myself as a writer. And that is true for many of the contributors to this book. However, there are experiences in everyone's life that cause us to "find our voice" and compel us to pause and reflect on how we got here and how it feels. Through these stories, I have found inspiration, humor and companionship – and I think you will too.

* * *

As I approached my 40th birthday, I sensed some major changes happening in this new decade of life. I had twenty years of experience at work behind me. My kids were no longer babies. And I felt more self-assured than ever, though without the cockiness of youth.

However, years of sunning in California were starting to leave lines on my face. My blond hair was showing signs of grey. There was no mistaking it – I was getting older.

Apparently this fact was not lost on the world around me. I had a "work crush" – you know, one of those secret little crushes on a co-worker that can keep work interesting but that you would never actually act on? My work crush was a 27-year-old cutie, and we got into some great conversations. After ten years of marriage with the same guy, it was fun to feel a little connection with someone new, someone unknown. Then one day he asks, "Do you like James Bond movies?" And I said, "Yes, I love James Bond," clearly seeing this as another point of commonality between my crush and me. And he said, "I knew you would. My Mom loves James Bond movies too." Ouch! Crushed by my crush.

It only got worse when I got an AARP card in the mail this year. It actually had *my* name on it. I checked because I thought it couldn't be – it must have been an old mailing list from when my Mom lived with us. But there it was – an AARP card with my name. I was shocked. Some delusional person had me confused with someone who is actually old. Not me! I called them up and made sure they understood that I was still closer to 30 than 60 and that I didn't need any more mailings from them for another two decades, thank you very much.

Despite a little moaning, I wasn't too worried about turning 40. I loved my life with a husband and children I adore, interesting friends who support me through thick and thin and a successful career. But approaching the likely halfway point of my life made me stop to take notice. Now was the time to ensure I was spending time on the right things and being true to myself. So maybe that's why there was change in the wind – maybe I had the confidence and security to feel the breeze and let it take me in new directions.

I talked to friends about life in their 40s. I started asking, "What is it like to be in your 40s?" to women at work, women in my Working Mothers Group, and moms at the soccer fields. What I found is that just about everyone had an opinion on the topic, usually a strong one. I expected many women to be concerned about being in their 40s. After all, weren't we on the cusp of giving up the physical allure that had given us some power over the years, whether we liked to admit it or not? It's harder to keep those few extra pounds off. We get fewer glances on the street from men. Sometimes it seems like my husband is getting more attractive to the opposite sex, while I'm getting less so.

We are at this "in-between" time. We are no longer "too young" for the Director or Vice President title at work. But we're starting to be "too old" to get pregnant, to be the young superstar at the office or to feel completely confident about the invincibility of our physical selves.

Just a few generations ago, for women born in the early 1900s, turning 40 meant being a first-time grandmother. Today, it often means being a first-time mom. Earlier, it meant heading into the final stretch of a woman's life when life expectancy was 50; today, it is the mid-way point of the current life expectancy of 80.[1]

Turning 40 is a milestone for women because, for many, it marks the end of our fertility. We're starting perimenopause. We see

[1] Source: National Vital Statistics System.

wrinkles, gain weight in parts of our body where our mothers did, make the decision to go grey, and lose our parents.

Ironically, our bodies may no longer want to bare children, but our minds offer fertile ground to develop other aspects of ourselves in our 40s. We have the experience, the confidence, and the perspective to make a significant difference at work, in our communities, and in our families. A new feeling of immediacy takes hold: "If this is something I want to do, I'd better do it now." If I'm going to have a kid, I'd better do it now. If I'm going to have the career I always wanted, I'd better start now. If I am going to have a happy marriage, I'd better dump this one now so I can start again.

And in fact, that's what I did. (Not dumping the marriage – I'm quite happy on that score). I had gotten the VP title, I was confident in my work and had a wide professional network and a strong record of achievements. But somehow it didn't matter quite as much. I lost the drive to prove myself at work. I realized that part of what had always driven me was proving to others that I was smart and competent. And proving to myself that I could support myself and my family, and didn't need to be financially dependent on anyone else. The notion of quitting work when I had children had been a frightening thought. What if something happened to my husband? What if he decided to end the marriage for some reason? I never wanted to be in a place financially where I had to make decisions based on my dependence on someone else. Ultimately, in addition to enjoying my job, the accolades and the opportunities, I was also staying out of fear that once I left the traditional workforce, I would never be able to get back in.

Once I turned 40, I somehow felt differently. I know it was really just one more day – that nothing had really changed that significantly. But I realized that the change I needed to make was to take a "career hiatus," to work on something new, develop new parts of myself.

So I quit my job, and decided to ask women to tell *their* story about life in their 40s. There were plenty of books written by experts about the physical and psychological changes women go through in their midlife. But nothing by "real" women on what they experienced, how they felt, and what they chose to do in this decade. I wasn't ready to read about menopause. Being in our 40s isn't just about what is going on physically. It's about the power and opportunities we have at this time in our lives. It's about our choices. It's about changes in relationships and changes in how we see ourselves.

* * *

By buying this book, you have supported the fight against breast cancer. I chose breast cancer as the benefit for this project because having our first mammogram marks the point of entry into this decade. Virtually all of us now have friends, colleagues, sisters and mothers who have battled breast cancer. The American Cancer Society reports that breast cancer incidence in women has increased from one in 20 in 1960 to one in eight today.[2] Every three minutes a woman in the United States is diagnosed with breast cancer.

Fortunately the survival statistics have improved significantly. Today a woman diagnosed with breast cancer has an 89% chance of surviving at least five years,[3] compared with 75% twenty years ago[4].

---

[2] American Cancer Society, Breast Cancer Facts & Figures 2007-2008.
[3] Ibid.
[4] National Cancer Institute, Annual Cancer Statistics Review, 1987.

Access to care and ongoing research are the two keys to continue this effort for our generation and for the generations of women to come.

For women just entering this decade, I hope this book will provide you with a glimpse into what's next, for yourself and your friends. For those already well along the journey, I hope you gain insights and perspective as you see elements of yourself or of other women you know. For all of us, I hope that this reflection on our own lives and our own Knowing Pains, past and future, will give us the strength to set our direction as a 40-something woman in today's world.

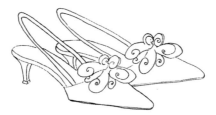

My Hair Experiment

By Natalie Serber

*R*ecently I decided I was tired of my gray roots. Why should I pay a small fortune every six weeks to disguise the truth of my age? I'm comfortable in my skin, I told myself. I'm a confident woman, my hair color isn't who I am, and this covering up is ridiculous, perhaps even weak. So began my *convincing myself* conversation.

On the one hand, I love sitting in the stylist's chair and having my head massaged, my hair smoothed and coifed in a way I'll never duplicate at home, listening to my stylist, Mimi, describe my new color as "delicious-rich-chocolaty-Italian-cinema-star-curvy." It makes me feel taller and sexier every time I leave the salon. On the other hand, in just a few short weeks the gray inches its way back. So I did the math. I thought about the social ramifications of coloring and what I was modeling to my children about aging and women and our society. And then decided it just wasn't worth it. I was woman enough to go gray. Would my family be so convinced?

"Dude-mom, at least wait until I'm in college," my seventeen-year-old son pleaded. I didn't think he'd even have an opinion.

"Mom, I totally get what you're doing," my fifteen-year-old daughter told me. "I think it's great and all. But just talking about it is enough. You don't actually have to, you know, *do it.*"

My husband tossed in "I love you no matter what," his usual non-committal response to anything regarding appearance. But I could tell he was doing the math, too.

Despite the mixed reviews, I told Mimi my plan, reasoning that to endure the gradual, growing thatch of gray roots was out of the question. She said, "You'll be daring, liberated." Then she grimly snipped the last evidence of my chemically-altered appearance. Mimi swung my salon-swivel chair for a full-mirror inspection. Wow, I never realized I had such a huge head! My pixie-cut was more Rosemary's Baby than cinema-star-curvy. In my new waxing-moon face, my wavering smile was lost. What had Mimi meant by liberated? Freed from the tyranny of the dye bottle or freed from prison camp?

Over the next weeks, I watched the gray fill in and I was horrified to discover how down-trodden I felt. Who knew I was so vain? What a great thing that I made myself go through this character-building change, I told myself in a self-help tone. Slowly I started to feel superior to my old self, like some strict-yet-generous, caftan-wearing spirit-guide telling the old me to "breathe."

Weeks went by and I blathered the story of my hair experiment to anyone who would listen – family, friends, neighbors, my barista, the grocery clerk, and my dry cleaner. I felt like I had to explain away my current physical state with my higher political/spiritual purpose. I was "embracing middle age."

And then, things turned really ugly. I began to feel superior to women my age who had obviously chosen to color. I'd see them at the coffee house or the library and I'd shake my sheep-shorn gray head, feeling sorry for their need to conform to our culture's youth adoration. "Poor things," I'd whisper to myself. "I feel sorry for you," I'd say, fueling my moral superiority while covering my staggering insecurity because they all looked Italian-cinema-fabulous. I was both bigger and smaller in exactly the same moment.

Of course, living with teenagers who are simultaneously hot and cold on any topic, I was used to quixotic emotions. My son, who had his first serious girlfriend (with astonishing lovely red hair), suddenly couldn't accommodate a mother and a true love at the same time. He just couldn't figure out how to make us both fit in his world. He let me know how inconsequential I'd become with the response to my hair queries, "Whatev."

My daughter was learning to live in her body in a new way, just as I was. Her shape blossomed, revealing burgeoning sexuality and confidence, while my knees and ass both withered. At one time, my broad shoulders seemed supple, now they felt tense with burden. She suggested that maybe I should give her all of my halter tops.

It was getting more difficult to support my hair color change. At some point, I just ended up feeling bad about myself on multiple levels. Not the least of which was emotional/intellectual. I was so petty! Clearly something had to change. My daughter gave me an out. "You know, Mom, you're not a cool person."

11

Great.

"I mean your skin looks better with warm tones."

I quizzed her further and she explained that my hair was not a generous silver, a cashmere-sweater gray or even a dove gray. My hair was manhole-cover gray. Does that make me an Autumn? I asked. She offered up a blank stare.

That was all it took. I called Mimi and she gasped, "Finally. Come in right now."

I have to confess, I adored the eye-watering moment of the first chemical whiff, the familiar sting of dye on my scalp. The full ninety minutes in the mysterious place that is a hair salon, the enigmatic land between before and after, where you exist totally in the moment, filled with the potential of what you might become.

My hair is now "flirty-mink-toasty-after-dinner-drink-luscious," according to Mimi. And I've learned to forgive myself for needing the boost. It's okay, I've decided, and it's relatively cheap after all. Hair dye is not the gateway drug to Botox and plastic surgery, not that there is anything wrong with those choices. My hair experiment made me a less judgmental brunette.

So now how do I deal with my roots? I go to Mimi more frequently. Will I go gray someday? Absolutely – perhaps when my daughter goes off to college with all my halter tops.

Natalie Serber (46) writes and teaches in Portland, Oregon where she lives with her husband and two children. Her work has appeared in *Inkwell Magazine, The Bellingham Review, Fourth Genre, Gulf Coast,* the collection, <u>Airfare: Stories, Poems and Essays on Flight</u>, and others. She is the recipient of the Tobias Wolff Award for Fiction and the John Steinbeck Award for Fiction, and has been short-listed for <u>Best American Stories</u>. Natalie is at work on a collection of linked stories, *Just be Glad I'm Your Mother*, and a novel with the working title *Boring, Oregon*. In the dark of night, Natalie has been known to post anonymous affirmative signs around her neighborhood just to spread a little goodwill.

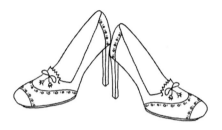

Full Cups

By Gabrielle Selz

For all those girls and women who long for big breasts, I was once one of you. I spent a good portion of my daydreaming life imagining and waiting to grow breasts. In my teens, while other girls' bosoms slowly (or in some cases quite rapidly) swelled, mine languished. I never grew out of an A-cup. In high school I was one of the girls in the locker room who was embarrassed because I never filled out the front of my gym uniform.

In my twenties, I wore undershirts that we called camisoles, but let's face it, they were just the small-breasted woman's attempt at sexy lingerie. I was thin and lithe, wiry and agile. I had lovely nipples and my breasts were actually rather beautifully shaped. And though they were small, my breasts were not ignored, at least not by men. My boyfriends said they loved them. They showered them with attention. But women were more critical. "You certainly won't fill out that dress, will you?" I've heard that more times than I care to remember. Or, "Oh, aren't they tiny and cute!"

For years I wanted a bosom. I wanted a fuller figure, a slope that filled out a sweater, a cleavage in which to dangle a locket. I wanted to have a pair of formidable breasts precede me into a room.

In my thirties, I was briefly married to a man who loved to photograph me naked. He told me I looked like a Greek Statue, a flying Nike. Yet as soon as we divorced, he married a woman who resembled me in all physical traits: tall, dark haired and leggy, except for her breasts. The girl was stacked.

"Oh, you're so lucky you don't have to wear a bra," my girlfriends exclaimed. If only I could find a bra, other than a stretchy, elastic sports bra, that fit me!

However, all that changed when I hit my 40s and got pregnant.

Suddenly I had what I'd desired and envied all those years – a full, growing bosom. As soon as I peed on the pregnancy test stick and saw my positive result, I ran out the door and hit the lingerie stores. I bought lacy bras in every color: black and red and dark navy with matching panties. I bought a pink bra with a little rose embroidered on the cups. I bought a leopard print bra and a wine-colored lace bra named The Moulin Rouge. I bought a bra of evergreen silk, in which my breasts nestled like two doves in a forest, and which I still have folded in my top drawer, because it's too beautiful to part with. I bought bras in different cup sizes, bustiers and racer-back bras. As my belly expanded, my breasts pumped up and my bra size grew. I sat on the beach six, seven and eight months pregnant in a bikini. Finally I had cleavage, and I wasn't going to waste it.

More than how it looked, I loved the way my breasts felt. They

15

felt delicious and soft and they rose like mounds of dough on my chest. Instead of the slender and limber girl I'd been, I suddenly felt as ripe and as plump as a summer melon. Finally, I knew what women meant when they called them, 'the girls.' I now had a pair of curvaceous girls of my own.

When my son was born, my milk came in with a vengeance. Whenever he cried, milk shot out of me spontaneously, like a fountain. Then I felt the full weight of my fertility. I felt fecund and like the earth itself, ready to feed. My breasts were the mountains that sat on this new landscape. I couldn't help it. I loved them. I loved the feel of them; the sudden and surprising heft of them. The way they jiggled and swung when I walked, the way they fell when I bent over, the way they sat upright in a bra or drooped to my sides when I lay in bed at night. I loved the way my contour – the line of my body, my topography, had changed.

I nursed solidly – my son never once sucked on a bottle or even a pacifier – for a year and a half. And though I loved my child nursing in my arms, wide eyed, staring up at me from where he feasted, mostly I just loved having those breasts.

Somehow I thought they'd stick around after the pregnancy, but they didn't. They deflated rapidly, more rapidly than they had inflated in fact, and my body went back to its willowy and flat-chested form.

I'm well into my forties now. I've considered implants, but my reasons against them are mostly tactile. How can you sleep on your stomach with a pair of implants, I wonder? If they don't fall to your sides, where do they go? I've felt other women's implants, touched and squeezed them, but nobody has ever told me, to my satisfaction, what they feel like from the inside.

This is, of course, the choice of someone who has not had breast cancer. My own little qualms about my small breasts seem downright frivolous when compared with women whose choices have been impelled by disease or disfigurement. Besides, what captivates me is my own body's capacity to, I guess, age. Because that's what growing means. It means to increase by size or addition. It means to expand, develop and become. What I've realized is that as I've aged, with or without big breasts, I've become more myself.

What I loved about my pregnant and nursing breasts was that they felt so much like me. They weren't perfect or symmetrical. When they were swollen with milk, they felt solid, full of the 'gravitas' of the mission at hand. But afterwards, when the nursing was done, they felt downright jovial and bouncy. Neither too big, nor too cumbersome, they were always in proportion and as agile as I was. I remember one summer night, right after my son was born, I was sitting outside with my husband as the fireflies danced. Our baby was asleep, wrapped in a blanket on the grass beside me. I was wearing a stretchy red dress. I'd worn this dress before, without breasts, but with breasts my body felt different, the dress felt different. The material clung to my breasts, my breasts pushed at the cloth, and it felt altogether sensual and alive. Without thinking I stood up and started cartwheeling across the lawn, spinning like a wheel, up and over, up and over. My dress flew over my head and suddenly my breasts were exposed to the cool night and bouncing upside down in the air like happy balloons. They made me laugh. I'll never forget how delicious that felt. How utterly abandoned and sexy it was to be me.

It's not that I don't feel sexy in my body anymore. I do, and more comfortable. This is my tool, my amazing vehicle. Most of what I feel, I feel first in my body. When I am anxious, my heart races. When I'm angry, I can feel the veins in my head expand as they become engorged with blood. When I'm happy I feel utterly light, and when I'm sad my body feels heavier, like there's more weight to cart around. Perhaps it took growing breasts for me to experience my body as the manifestation of my emotional landscape and my changing journey through life. Other woman may experience different parts of their body changing and maturing, but this is where I learned, in a real sense, that how I experience myself is how others experience me. And when I walk with confidence into a room, with or without a formidable bosom preceding me, people can tell.

I see women now who are slightly ahead of me in age. They're in their fifties, and they've begun to inhabit their bodies differently. It's as if they've taken root inside themselves and they sit and move with grace and confidence. I want to grow into and become one of these women, planted firmly in my own body, a body that changes over time. Maybe when I hit menopause I'll grow breasts again. It's not that unlikely – I've known women who have suddenly become rather well-endowed as they go through their change of life. In the meantime, I have my willowy, agile body, I have my health, I have my deliciously small breasts.

Here's what I would tell someone younger, who longs, as I once did, for a C-cup. Enjoy everything you have while you have it. Admire yourself. Wear the bikini anyway. Grow into yourself. Your body will change over time. You have no idea what surprises are in store for you. If I'd always had breasts, the novelty of my pregnant and nursing breasts would never have thrilled me as they did. Most likely I would have spent a good deal of time complaining about my weight gain and sagging flesh. But I celebrated my changing body. I want to remember that as I ripen. I want to move forward in wonder at my body's capacity, its elasticity, and its growth. Here it is. It is so wonderful now. I should never complain. There's no hurry. The thin girl I once was is now an elegant woman.

Gabrielle Selz (48) is a freelance writer living in Southampton, New York with her awesome son Theo and her feisty little dog, Rufi. She has worked in commercial and children's television, and like many city dwellers, she hardly ever saw daylight until fleeing the city to fulfill her need to see the horizon. She grew up bicoastal in both the New York and the Berkeley bohemian art worlds of the 60s and 70s, where huge appetites and wild imaginations were the norm. Her work has appeared in publications such as *MORE, Newsday,* online at ducts.org and in *The New York Times.* Currently she's writing a memoir and compiling a history about the utopian artist housing project, Westbeth.

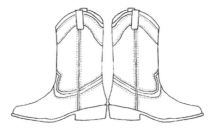

I Declare

By Diane Perro

I declare 2000: *The Year of Cleavage!*" I shouted as my girlfriends and I raised champagne to toast the New Millennium, and fireworks exploded over the San Francisco Bay.

Years ago, I gave up making New Years *resolutions* in favor of *declarations*. A declaration carries strength and authority. It's also much easier to keep. Consider the typical list of resolutions: lose 20 pounds, exercise every day, improve finances, learn something new, do whatever it is you've had on the list for the past 15 years but still haven't done. Talk about a recipe for disappointment and guilt. I used to write down the same things year after year, never keeping my promises. Not anymore. I want to keep my promises, and now I try to set reasonable, achievable goals – preferably ones that I enjoy accomplishing.

During *The Year of Being Good to Myself,* I took an exotic 3-week vacation, had a mani/pedi every other week, massages once a month, and as many facials as I could tolerate. In *The Year of Finding a Good Man,* I found many good men, had many good dates, and considered the year a total success, unlike one of my friends who had resolved to find *the* good man (of her dreams) and had failed miserably, often drowning her sorrows with her favorite *two* good men, Ben and Jerry.

You may think I sound like a spokesperson for some underachiever advocacy group. But I've made some fairly impressive achievements in my life, like becoming the director of an inner-city gospel choir when I was only 19, managing a successful multi-million dollar international conference, biking to the top of a volcano, and coming to peace with my thighs. It wasn't easy. I'd hated my thighs since I was a 6th grader trying to stuff myself into Levi's, the jean du jour, which back then only came in slim-cut male sizes. I'd spent nearly 20 years trying to hide my thighs or squeeze them into the latest fashions, avoiding any invitations that involved wearing a bathing suit in mixed company. But at some point in my early thirties, I finally took a good long look at my thighs. I saw that they are bigger than average, always would be, and they'll never be suitable for miniskirts or skinny boy-cut jeans. I also noticed that they are strong, devoid of saddlebags, and nicely balance out my rather bountiful bosom. So I declared a truce. And my thighs and I have coexisted harmoniously ever since.

The Year of Cleavage was a complete success. In addition to the four of us on the waterfront that New Year's Eve, many of our girlfriends later joined the movement. Cleavage was shown worldwide from San Francisco to Bali as we all made a conscious effort to "display the girls" whenever appropriate. And as necklines plunged, our popularity skyrocketed. Men fell all over themselves to open our doors, buy our drinks and generally get to know us. We couldn't have been more popular that year if we'd been handing out free beer. Some of us even ventured onto beaches topless during vacations to Europe and Indonesia. It was liberating, empowering, and not the least bit painful thanks to SPF45 waterproof sunscreen. As 2000 was drawing to a close, I would make another declaration, one that I had no real intention of keeping, but one that, along with other unforeseen events, would change my life forever.

It was Election Day. I was visiting a friend in Hong Kong and asked if he would turn on CNN so we could check the results. We discovered that it was as yet undecided but it was down to Florida where there was some discrepancy with the count. I was both horrified and appalled. "If George Bush becomes President, I'm moving to Paris!" I declared. It just flew out of my mouth.

But a month later as the year came to a close, I'd forgotten all about this unwitting declaration and was fixated on a single thought. Obsessed, I could only think to declare 2001 as *The Year I Turn 40.* Forty. God, that sounded old. But I didn't *feel* old. Didn't really look that old either. I wondered what turning 40 would feel like, what it would mean to me, but I hadn't a clue. Would 40 be the peak? Would it all be downhill (and not the good kind of downhill) from there? I had a lot of questions, but no answers.

I didn't realize then that 2001 would also be *The Year One of My Best Friends Would Die in a Plane Crash.* I didn't realize that it would be a year that would make me question almost everything, and a year that would give me few answers.

Nobody will ever forget the events that took place that day in September. I certainly don't need to be reminded. While I recognize September 11th for its national - even global - significance, for me it's very personal. It's the day that I lost someone I loved dearly. It's the day my friend Tommy died.

A week after September 11th, still in shock, I found myself at the White House with Tommy's family and the other families of the victims of United Flight 93. We were invited to receive condolences and a personal thank you from the President, First Lady, and the entire White House staff for our loved ones, whose acts of bravery kept Flight 93 from hitting its target. There I was, being ushered from one differently colored room to the next until I stood face-to-face with the man that I had been bad-mouthing. The President of our country took my hand, looked into my eyes, kissed me on the cheek and said, "I'm sorry about your friend." Moments later that same man was waving his arm and calling to me, "Yeah, come on, Di. Come and get in the picture! Come on, Di!" I hustled across the room to stand alongside Tommy's family as an aide took a picture of us with President Bush and the First Lady. Surreal doesn't begin to describe it. Despite my feelings for George W. Bush, that day I felt no animosity for him or anyone. I couldn't feel much of anything, except confusion and profound sadness.

I was utterly disillusioned, and the days that followed were a blur. I spent a lot of time sitting on my horse Cody, riding trails along the beautiful hills that overlook the Pacific Ocean. I thought about everything that had happened and was continuing to happen, often with tears streaming down my face. Had the world gone mad? What could I expect for the future? Is it going to get worse? Why Tommy?

23

Why couldn't I have met President Clinton instead of Bush? Did I get another case of poison oak, or are my allergies just acting up again?

Honestly, at some point I just got tired of crying and wondering and asking myself questions that I simply couldn't answer. More and more I began to ask myself questions that I could answer (or that just gave me a much needed giggle). Slowly, my mind began filling with normal, everyday thoughts again. As it turned out, I didn't have another case of poison oak, but I did have an itch to live my life more fully. I desperately wanted to find normal again. I was pretty sure that if I kept looking hard enough, eventually I would find it. And I'd rediscover that good humored, somewhat irreverent, go-for-it gal that I'd always been.

The Year I Turn 40 had taken an unexpected turn. Our country had suffered a horrific event that killed my friend and many others. Some nut case was sending Anthrax-grams, and our government had started a war in Afghanistan. As my birthday approached, I realized that if I didn't do something, *The Year I Turn 40* would be completely overshadowed by death, insanity and sorrow.

I thought back to that declaration I had made in the heat of the moment during the election, the one I'd just blurted out. Well, why not? Thank goodness my two best friends are spontaneous travelers. With little notice, we flew to Paris. So it wasn't a move but it was a fabulous vacation and a great way to celebrate my 40th birthday.

Returning from my trip, I felt revitalized. My world was bright and positive again. But as the weeks and months wore on, that feeling started to wear thin. It wasn't just the weight of the world's events or the death of my friend. It was me. It was my life that was weighing me down. And as I sat in my office one day staring at my laptop, I realized that I would rather drive a large stake through the middle of my forehead than continue doing what I was doing. I had worked in technology for about fifteen years, going from one company and marketing job to the next, and I just couldn't do it any more. I needed a change. A *big* one. And I knew what I had to do. Make good on that promise – really move to Paris.

Could I do it? To ensure that I would stick to my plan, I told all of my friends that I was moving. I had no idea what was in store for me, and some days I wondered why I was planning to leave a city and friends I loved. But most days I just knew that I was doing something I needed to do. And that was all I needed to know.

Some say it takes a village, and let me tell you, to move me from San Francisco to Paris, it did. My parents flew in from Minnesota to help me sell most of my belongings. Friends still laugh about my mother's practical Midwestern pricing (ironing board: $20, vintage McCoy vase: 50 cents) and her keen bargaining skills honed by years of staging and frequenting garage sales. Despite my mother's fear of having her only daughter miles away, living in a country that didn't even *like* Americans from what she'd heard, as we stood taking one last look at my empty apartment she hugged me and said, "You have to do what makes you happy." My father was vicariously excited for me. He is, like his daughter, prone to wanderlust. But I knew he was a bit worried, too. So was I. What did I think I was going to do in Paris, where I had no job, no friends, and no plan? But had I waited for a plan, I would still be waiting.

From the instant I landed in Paris, I knew I was where I was meant to be. As I walked around the Jardin du Luxembourg that first day, I felt a joy and a freedom that I hadn't felt in years. I was overwhelmed with the excitement of the unknown and a magnificent feeling of lightness. I had kept my promise. I was living in Paris.

It hasn't always been easy. The language and culture are a constant struggle, looking for apartments was painful, and trying to get cable installed proved impossible. Even doing something as simple as signing up for French courses made me want to pull out my hair. (I have to confess that instead of pulling out my hair, I went to a lingerie shop and spent my tuition on new bras with matching panties. I really can't explain why, in my frustration, I did this. But every time I've recounted this story to a French woman, she has applauded me and said that the money was well spent because everyone knows that the way to learn French is to find yourself a French lover, and sexy lingerie is a *must* for that!)

I can't say that I've mastered the language yet, nor have I learned to completely navigate the culture. But what I *have* learned is how to slow down, do less, and enjoy more. How to appreciate life, my friends, and my family more than ever. Though I can still be as impractical as I ever was, I have learned that I can live a simpler life and be even happier. I've always believed that a person needs to get outside their comfort zone to find out who they really are, and what they really want out of life. Paris has certainly been way outside my comfort zone at times and it's wonderful to know that, at the halfway point in my life, there's still more to learn and discover.

I have been living in Paris for over five years and it has been a wild ride. I've made many wonderful new friends and am thankful that many of my old friends have visited numerous times (though I didn't really have to twist their arms). I spent the first two years living a crazy Bohemian life singing, writing, traveling, designing, and hanging out in smoky bars and cafes until all hours. Eventually my diminishing savings account and conservative midwest work ethic got the better of me, and I took a *real* job that has taken me back, ironically, to San Francisco. So for the past year, I've been splitting my time between the two cities I love. And I have to pinch myself.

I'm not sure what I'll declare for next year. Haven't a clue. But I know that whatever it is, it will be something positive and achievable. And I'll make good on my promise.

Diane Perro (46) is a marketing specialist who has helped brand and launch several high-tech startups. Not one to be defined by a single career, Diane has lent her marketing talents to the non-profit world and tried her semi-professional hand as a costumier, seamstress, florist, and singer-songwriter—spanning gospel to rock. Her varied endeavors have resulted in myriad experiences that she has chronicled and hopes to publish one day as a collection of essays. Meanwhile she loves living in the land of brie, croissants and great lingerie.

Fanning the Flames of Youth

By Nancy Davis Kho

ometimes, when I'm standing in line at the grocery store with my basket full of free-radical fighting blueberries, iron-rich lentils and tasteless fiber crackers, I look at the newsstand headlines and sigh in near-defeat. The glossy mags are full of breaking news stories aimed at women younger than I who still have a chance to capture and preserve the youthfulness that is, even now, draining out of their pores while they stand listening to the beeping of the barcode scanner. Could it be that I squandered the past two decades establishing my career and raising two young children, when I should have spent more time clutching at the youth that the media tells us is so eminently desirable?

And then, a song comes over the in-store Muzak system – a tinny, knock-off version of a song to be sure, but one that I recognize. My forehead smooths, I stand up straight and lose an inch off my spare tire, and my hair grows naturally blond. It's "Something So Strong" by Crowded House.

You see, it would probably be too late for me to avoid an express ticket to Old Lady Land, wrinkled tissue and cavernous handbag in hand, were it not for one practice I took up at age 14, and have been following faithfully ever since:

I am a fan of rock musician Neil Finn.

Neil fronted the eclectic art rock band Split Enz in the 1970s, then went on to form Crowded House in the '80s. After the band broke up in 1996, Neil did solo albums and toured with his brother Tim. He is often cited as "the songwriter's songwriter," turning out genius melodies that skilled musicians envy, but that are generally underappreciated by the world at large. Neil's music is sprinkled with instruments not often found in rock music, like the ukulele and violin. His songs boast soaring harmonies, fascinating lyrical juxtapositions, and catchy hooks that linger in the listener's head. Neil's great stage patter and rugged good looks, with a boyish forelock of hair just now going grey, are merely a bonus.

Now, I don't claim that Neil Finn's music has magical, youth-restoring powers. Rather, it's the act of being a devoted rock fan that has had such positive, healthful effects. I have quite a few friends who swear by the Dave Matthews version of this treatment, and a beloved sister-in-law whose bell rings for Barry Manilow.

The restorative effects of such attachment are not limited to music fans, of course. That commitment could be to anything, from bass fishing to knitting to pole vaulting. What I've learned is that embracing the passion, evolving and changing along with it over the years, can be powerful medicine.

For example, speaking from my own experience, there are myriad tangible ways in which being a rock fan keeps a person young. Staying current with new music releases requires cutting-edge technological savvy. I bought my first Neil Finn music on vinyl when I was fourteen; his latest was downloaded to my laptop via a wireless connection and then transferred to my iPod. In order to stay abreast of his new projects, I, like Neil, have progressed from vinyl, to cassette, to CD, and now to digital downloading. Last weekend I spent an hour optimizing the media player on my laptop to watch a live Crowded House studio session, thereby adding another notch to my tech-support belt on behalf of the man from New Zealand. I challenge any twenty-year-old to download a song faster than I do. Neil may be the reason I someday learn to text message.

Being a fan also provides a more compelling incentive for good health than any of the aging studies I've read in self-help magazines. Every two or three years, Neil tours with his band, including a visit to my town. That means it's time to suck in my gut and put on my good concert jeans, high heeled boots and a shirt that communicates devotion just short of stalking. One never knows at which show one will *finally* be pulled onstage to sing along, or play ukulele, and one must be prepared. I have only to picture that magic moment as my Pilates instructor yells, "Four more! Three more! Two more!" and I can dispel the image of my beating her senseless with a hand weight.

Good physical conditioning is also a prerequisite for the sprint to the stage that invariably precedes Neil's concerts. As the lights dim for the musicians to take the floor, I float like a butterfly and sting like a bee to the front-most position I can secure. A friend of mine who once accompanied me to one of his shows still shakes her head at the memory of my saying, "I'm just gonna try to…" and then disappearing for the rest of the evening as I fought to a position at the front of the stage. In my defense, my friend is younger than I, and I assumed she was following in my wake.

A commitment to a particular musician can also keep reflexes sharp, which, as any medical professional will say, is a hallmark of youthfulness. Two years ago, Neil and brother Tim were scheduled to play at a local concert hall. One of the radio stations in town offered up the chance for fifteen lucky listeners to attend a private concert with The Finn Brothers. To win, you just had to be caller number twelve whenever a Finn Brothers song was played.

When the contest week started, my reflexes were good – too good. Twice, I was caller two, and twice I was caller five. By the final opportunity to win, I had perfected my delayed response so that I was caller eleven. That's right, the very next caller after me got the final set of tickets. I feel certain that one additional chance would have seen me in the winner's circle, holding a ticket to the private concert, rather than sitting on the kitchen floor weeping while my children looked on in curiosity.

Rock fans often form and maintain community connections as a consequence of their devotion. This is important, because research has shown that people with strong social networks live longer and healthier lives.

I finally realized at forty that I was confident enough to do something for which I lacked the courage when I was younger: I joined the Neil fan forum on the Internet. Many times each day members of the community, better known as Frenz, post burning topics such as

"Neil's Approach to Tonality" or "Who's a better musician, Neil or Tim Finn?" Posters are guaranteed an immediate response from a small and devoted band of followers like Half-Full and Texas Rose. It makes me feel better to know that there are others like me out there, burnishing our devotion in obscurity.

I know I will never be lonely while Frenz roam the Internet, and the land, with FINN printed in permanent black marker on the back of their hands at the appointed "Meet Up" spot prior to each of his shows.

Although an artist as talented as Neil is winning new fans with each fresh project, it's an undeniable fact that the fan base and the artist alike are aging. One of the topics on the Frenz board that drew the most response during his last U.S. concert tour was whether Neil was wearing orthopedic shoes onstage. I understand the impulse that drove so many people to reflect on the subject. If the object of our affection is wearing orthopedic shoes…does that mean we're old enough for them too?

The first time I saw Neil live in concert was when I was in college in the '80s. It was a long subway ride through a dicey part of Philadelphia to get there, and the venue was somewhat rundown. Once inside, the place hummed with energy, as Neil and his band ripped through hits from their latest album. No one sat. Everyone crushed towards the stage and danced.

The last time I saw Neil play live, it was in a concert hall with thick, cushioned red velvet seats that rocked comfortably – no need to rush the stage – and a wine bar in the lobby. The show was musically as good as anything I'd heard him play, but the crowd's energy was unquestionably sedate.

I brought along a friend who'd never heard Neil play live, and I found myself apologizing for what I perceived as a lack of oomph. "There's usually so much more crowd excitement than this! We're usually all dancing and singing along!" My friend laughed and told me he loved the show and that he recognized Neil's musical genius.

And that's when it hit me. Orthopedic shoes, rocking chairs and all; we may be getting older, but the inner flame of passion burns as brightly as ever. Maybe it even blazes a bit higher these days, as we fans raise the next generation of devotees. Our two daughters, who as infants rocked to sleep while I sang them Neil's "Message to My Girl," are crazy about his music. When our oldest daughter was five she made me a sign to carry to a concert; written in shaky crayon on a piece of construction paper was the word ENCROE.

Neil Finn may not be your cup of tea, but I hope something is. Something that gives you the same feeling inside as it did the first time you discovered it, that eternal thrill of excitement and affinity and reward.

And I warn you: if you are standing between Neil Finn and me when he plays at my nursing home someday, step aside. You do *not* want to be in my way.

Nancy Davis Kho (42) is a writer based in the San Francisco Bay Area. She is a frequent contributor to the San Francisco Chronicle, and her essays and articles have also appeared in publications including Pink Magazine, Adirondack Life, and CommonSenseMedia.org. She is the author of *The Second Mrs. Douglass,* a novel to be published in 2009. Shortly after writing the essay that appears in this book, she met musician Neil Finn, who complimented her on her fake New Zealand accent.

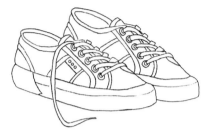

The Real Marathon

By Tina Goette

*A*ccording to my 4-year-old daughter, I'm 71 years old (that's the word she spread at her preschool on my 41st birthday). Admittedly, there are many days when I think I know what it feels like to be 71.

Apparently, I'm also under some misguided impression that I'm a runner. At least, I'm desperately trying to convince myself that I'm a runner. As the coordinator for San Francisco's physical activity and healthy eating initiative, I've got to practice what I preach…so I signed on to run the San Francisco Half Marathon.

It was December, and I was newly divorced and eight months into my 40s, when I decided I should take this Shape Up Challenge. I outfitted myself with a Craigslist jog stroller and off we went for my inaugural run. At the half mile marker (five whole city blocks), I had to bend over and breathe deeply to avoid passing out. I started up again, only to stop two blocks later to repeat. My daughter, a keen observer, goaded, "Mommy, why did you stop running? Keep going!" "Okay coach," I muttered under my breath, only to turn back at the next possible juncture to end the misery. At this rate, it would surely be a long, hellacious trip.

That Christmas was my first as a divorcée, the first Christmas I had to share my sweet girl with her father on what had always been a cherished family celebration, both in marriage and before. It was something of a watershed event for me (and yes, I cried). On that Christmas Day, I thought I'd embrace the Jewish "tradition" of going to the movies on Christmas, while my babe was with her father. I enjoyed the idea that I'd go alone and celebrate my singlehood, and revel in my newfound freedom and happiness. When I arrived at the movie theater, it was closed. It felt like a cruel joke. So I went home, laced my shoes and went for a jog, figuring what better gift to give myself than health. This time I made it seven blocks before the wheezing set in... asthma... what a perfect topper to my first Christmas alone. I walked home and, as I was closing the door, the phone rang. It was the ex, he was done, and wanted to see whether he could bring my daughter home early. There was the gift I'd been waiting for.

This story is about ME, not about him. But our lives are now inextricably intertwined. He is a part of me, not only through our daughter, but by virtue of the fact that our union had me thoroughly questioning my sanity, my ability to make good choices, and my friendships. It left me wondering whether I could ever trust or love another man again. After waiting for 36 years to get married, the one I chose turned out to be the polar opposite of everything he claimed to be; this truth slowly revealing itself over time, beginning shortly after our wedding. After three years of explaining away my ex's bad behavior, I stopped justifying it and called it as I saw it. I did my homework, pored obsessively over my budget, consulted an attorney, and warned friends and family what was in the offing. A sucker for symbolic gestures, I ended it on Friday the 13th. And that's enough ink on him.

I started running in earnest in January. My Saturday mornings, when my daughter was with her dad, were the dedicated training days. I held them holy, disallowing any distractions (including the occasional hangover, foot injury, etc.) to keep me from my regimen. As the weeks passed, I noticed how my calves tightened, and my bottom lifted. I was feeling goooood.

The SF Marathon folks earnestly advised that I needed to put more miles in during the week, that I should follow their training program. All I could think was, "Great, more guilt" for all the times I wouldn't be able to follow the program and go for those other two, progressively longer, midweek runs. So I did the best I could: Saturday mornings with occasional bonus runs.

Living in San Francisco, it became my mission to find the flattest possible training route (never mind that the actual marathon course itself was littered with hills). When I discovered it, I wore down the pavement on that 1.3 mile loop.... Over time, I'd add a mile or two to my total distance, finding it stunning that three months ago I couldn't run a mile, and I was now up to a whole five miles – *without stopping*. But I also couldn't fathom the concept that at five miles I was just over a third of the way there with four months to go. And the drum beat on... "How on earth will I ever do this? WHY am I attempting this?"

The tempo remained steady through winter and spring. I grew stronger, my stamina deepened, my confidence blossomed. I found myself brushing away trivial irritations at the office. When the ex didn't show, or committed some other nonsense, I shrugged my shoulders and rolled with it. I started to enjoy my Saturday morning runs. I also finally had the confidence to break away from my "flattest route in the neighborhood" path and start doing hills.

Yes, I did have that jog stroller, which I occasionally put to use on those odd weekday mornings. I was judicious with it when I realized just how much harder it is to run when you're pushing an extra 40 pounds (which of course made me wonder just how much easier this whole exercise would be if I simply were 40 pounds lighter).

Then, in June, the ex stopped showing up for my daughter. My Saturdays no longer consisted of leisurely, fulfilling runs with my friends, but solo runs of necessity (while pushing that extra 40 pounds, uphill, both ways …in the snow). Saturday mornings were now hectic, testing my patience at every turn as I urged my daughter to get up, eat, dress, brush teeth, brush hair, so I could run her to her dance class. On the upside, by the time we got out the door, I didn't even realize I was running, I was so busy responding to the constant chatter of my passenger.

In this fashion, for several weeks, I cobbled together runs building up to seven miles. I was proud of myself, but still a bit worried that I hadn't yet hit the 10 mile mark that 'those who know' say is the minimum you should run prior to taking on a half marathon. I had three weeks left, and figured I still had time to get there. At least, until I talked to another expert a week later who responded to my weekend plans with, "You're going for a long run? Aren't you supposed to be tapering, letting those legs get good and rested?" Ugh, a hit to the solar plexus… I wasn't going to get to 10 miles. He was right. I had to rest. Would I, could I, make it on seven miles?

As the race neared, I did a few workouts to remind my muscles of their looming responsibilities. I also grew increasingly fatalistic as each day passed. The invariable question, "Are you ready?" was met with a nervous laugh, wave of my hand, and an unsure "Sure!"

And suddenly it was July 29: The San Francisco Marathon. A date I regarded with fear and some level of loathing. How could I possibly run 13.1 miles if the longest distance I'd managed over the course of eight long months was seven? I'd told far too many people what I was attempting. I couldn't back out. I couldn't walk away without even trying… I needed a success – whether or not I finished. I needed to say I had tried.

When the gun sounded, off I went, alone, amidst thousands of other would-be half marathoners, a familiar mantra replaying, "How the heck did I get myself into this? Can I do it? How will I ever make it?"

I found myself crying as I set off across the starting line. And when I envisioned myself crossing the finish line the tears flowed with still greater force. I was embarrassed to be crying, but couldn't help myself: I was proud just for being there.

When I finally got those emotions under control, I focused on my race strategy. I promised myself that no matter what happened, I would run at least seven miles before I could start walking, because I knew I could do at least that. At mile three, I wondered how I'd ever get to mile seven, let alone 13; the blisters were forming. San Francisco is small – it's only 7 x 7 miles… so to map out a marathon, they had us running switchbacks… tempting me to cross over to the (dark) side where the runners were returning from the place I had yet to go, but I stayed on my side.

As I ran, I recounted the past year, but mostly the last few months. Amidst my ex's absence was upheaval. He'd quit his job, had no phone, got into trouble, found a new girlfriend… In response, I had reverted to my marital days as spy and detective. I dissected his every word, obsessing about which part of his stories was fact and which was fiction. It occurred to me that the last couple of months I had been living HIS life, not MINE. I had allowed his drama to create havoc in my life, as well as bitterness, fear and resentment.

That is the real marathon, where stamina is a constant and the mental game is the one I need to conquer. My training proved that I can push through the physical pain, and conquer the mind games to convince my body that it actually enjoys running. All I needed to do now was to apply that mental resolve to my new role as a divorcee and single mother. It was there, with that realization and at mile five when I noticed, "I can do this, I feel good."

Over 2½ hours later, at 12.9 miles, I started looking for my cheerleaders. My delusion of grandeur to cross the finish line before thousands of adoring fans was shattered as there were few spectators left. I ran over to my personal fan club for hugs, kisses, and pictures; then hobbled on across the finish line for a 2:52:08 finish. My daughter, still clutching her "Go, Mommy, Go!" sign, ran into my arms screaming "Good job, Mommy!"

Looking back, my half marathon goal was quite audacious. On one hand, it was audacious in what it lacked. It required tuning out the experts and training the only way that worked for my life, my schedule, my sanity, and my daughter. On the other hand, it was audacious in what it represented: hope, belief and sheer willpower. What I lacked in youthful vigor, I made up for in determination, humility and community. I had to ask for help from friends, family and my daughter. In my youth, I lacked the audacity to even consider, let alone accept, such a challenge. In my forties, I just went for it because getting divorced was simply the first step in my marathon toward creating a newly confident, happy and audacious me.

Tina Goette (41) is a public health professional for the City of San Francisco's Department of Public Health. She coordinates the City's chronic disease prevention efforts through the Shape Up SF Initiative. Tina walks the talk by "Escaping from Alcatraz" in the icy waters of San Francisco Bay, and recently completed the San Francisco Marathon. Tina is a frequent speaker and a published author in peer-reviewed journals and public health textbooks. In addition to her professional writings, Tina gained a following of family, friends, and friends of friends with her monthly *Dating Chronicles* in 2001. As a single mom, she is devoted to raising a thoughtful, kind, inquisitive and spunky daughter.

Answering the Call

By Elizabeth Becker

When I was halfway through high school, I got a feeling. Well, actually I got several feelings in high school – but this is not the story of my sexual awakening, or my misguided attempts to prove myself worthy by being a remarkable student.

No, this story is about experiencing a particular feeling that was quiet, unwelcome, confusing, and unrelenting. And how that feeling persisted for years – over 25 years – until, as I turned 40, I realized that I needed to face this feeling once and for all - or risk dying without fully realizing my potential.

You see, I was experiencing a "spiritual calling." Trouble was, I didn't know it was a "spiritual call" and I did not really want this particular call – or rather, I was not sure what to do with it. All I knew was that my life was statistically nearly half over and I felt that I wasn't doing the one thing that I knew I was supposed to be doing.

I'm getting ahead of myself. I'll start back a few years and you'll see what I mean.

When I was 15 years old, I was a nice Roman Catholic girl attending a private all-girls prep school in suburban Philadelphia. So when I got this strange feeling, I *knew*, as only a teenager could know with complete certainty, that it was the call that I had been prepared for, taught to look for, it was… (Cue baritone "radio voice") GOD CALLING.

That year, I came face to face with the fact that I had what I then *knew* was a "religious" calling. Generally, being a young woman with a religious calling is not a great thing by society's standards. As a Roman Catholic – it really could not get any worse. As I saw it, there was only one career path for young women with a religious calling. I was certain that I was being called to be a nun. That's right – no sex, bad clothes, poverty, and god-forbid – obedience. Yikes! Was there any upside? At least if I'd been born Protestant, I could have had a few chances to become a minister or a priest. Not so with the Catholics – women are out of any of the top jobs.

I remember lying awake in bed and thinking about how I was the one to cry at all the hymns at Mass. Was I really the only one with a call? Why did the stories of the Bible speak to me? Did others seem to get a secret message too?

I would spend the last few minutes of every day praying for some other call – anything. Perhaps a call to the legal profession, becoming a veterinarian, or even to the harsh duty of marrying a millionaire and managing a family fortune. Anything else, dear Lord, hear my prayer. Oh, *please*.

I waged an internal battle with myself and my God. Could I

really be "Sister Elizabeth," "Sister Liz"? Could I give up having a husband, children, a beach house? (In those years, I saw having a beach house on the Jersey Shore as the ultimate payoff for a successful career or marrying well.) How much did I really love God? Enough for this? Did God really mean me, or was I mistakenly intercepting the call for the girl who sat behind me in homeroom who seemed way more pious? I even questioned if there really was a God, or if I was just experiencing some neurosis or undocumented side-effect of puberty.

I kept asking God, *Really?* and *Are you sure you mean me?* God's answer was always, *Yes* and then something more… but nothing clear. Who knew that God mumbled…

For the next few years, I became obsessed with nuns – old ones, fat ones and especially the new ones – the novitiates who looked so earnest and stiff. I pondered about the Sister who taught at my high school who seemed too pretty to be a nun. What *happened to her?* I wondered. *How did she know?* I watched nuns at Mass, studied how they talked and lived together. I even went out of my way one cold winter day to watch them sledding on the "mother-house hill" with their blue dresses flapping ridiculously in the wind.

Then after a while I realized I had a *big* problem with my call. I found that indeed God *was* listening to my prayers. For every time I would get ready to dance the "Liz as a nun" dance with God, the music would stop.

I realized that, Yes, I did have a call, but No, it was not to become a nun. "But that's all I know," I screamed at God one afternoon from the beach after senior year. "What do you want from me?" I was frustrated and angry. I felt like a betrayed girlfriend who was suffering by the phone. Oh God called alright, but always hung up as soon as I picked up the receiver.

While in college, I tried going to Mass. However, I became increasingly resentful of the Roman Catholic Church which, as an institution, did not seem to be open to women serving in equal ways to men. Eventually I stopped going to church, as it seemed contradictory to be attending church while fundamentally disagreeing with the leadership. I announced to my very conservative father that I no longer considered myself a Catholic. I think I broke his heart. I still believed in God but I stopped practicing my faith.

I also gave up on ever trying to understand this "calling." But God did not give up on me. He kept calling.

Rrring, rrring,

Hello?

Click.

God, damn it. You again.

So for over 20 years I stayed in that place – angry and aware, cranky and stupidly hopeful, still hearing the call, knowing that God was there, but without an answer for me. I often felt abandoned by God who would not give me the answers.

During those years, I found that I missed going to church. I would visit a Mass and feel empty, divorced from God – like I used to be part of the family, but was not really at home there anymore. I tried other Christian denominations, visited a Jewish temple and even studied Buddhism. I felt sad that I couldn't find a place to practice my faith that felt like a fit. So while I still believed in God and felt God's presence in my life, I didn't have a spiritual practice for years. I felt adrift and unfulfilled.

Meanwhile, I am happy to say that I did figure out a few other things. I found peace in my yoga practice. I liked to run and bike. I was a strong leader who could lead global teams in large organizations. I realized that I could not make a flaky-perfect pie crust like my grandmother did and, more importantly, I did not care as I thought I should. I learned that I could love and be loved deeply. I found out that I was impatient with details. I found I could overcome my fears of becoming a mother, and gave birth to two beautiful children. I learned that I am an instigator, a creator and a visionary.

And I learned that this feeling, this call, was real and was not going away. What I still could not learn, though, was what I was supposed to do with it.

Right around the time I turned 40 two things happened: I became pregnant with our second child and my employer and I decided to part company. Because I now had some extra time on my hands, I could finally slow down long enough to spend some time with the incessant calling. I decided that instead of running from the call as I had since college, I would turn my face to the call and meet it head on. I was determined not to wonder at my death what would have happened if I had only followed my call.

That summer I attended a spiritual workshop where I finally had a breakthrough. It came during a walking meditation within an open spiral labyrinth while considering some words from a Rainer Maria Rilke letter. The words were like God finally speaking clearly to me. Tears of relief and joy ran down my face as these words told me to be patient with things that were unanswered in my heart. The message challenged me to love the questions, not to look for the answers, and to try to experience everything. It suggested that if I lived my life experiencing the questions, perhaps someday I would experience the answers. Ahh, finally a message that I could understand.

As I walked, I realized that instead of having a "religious calling," one that called me to be a nun or minister, I was having a "spiritual calling," one less defined or exacting. I also realized that, instead of turning away from God because I could not discern His message, I could stay present. I would live the question, walk with the question, and stand, holding the question. The answer was not in testily slamming down the receiver when no one responded. It was in keeping the line open.

So I started standing, walking, being. "I am called," I would repeat. "No, I have not yet figured it out, but that's okay." Where I had once been angry and closed, I became open and willing to just live there. No running, no expletives, no griping. Just, "I am called."

I bought some books on what I came to learn was called "discernment" – some were helpful, some were not. I sat down with a minister at my neighborhood church and spilled out the whole story. He asked me if he could pray for me. This gesture and his prayer moved me to tears. I knew I was doing the right thing. I visited the local seminary and decided not to go – at least not yet. I finally shared all of this "calling stuff" with my husband who was also raised Roman Catholic. He was a little confounded: "What are you going to be? The next Mother Teresa? The minister at the local church?" he asked. I stood with that too. "I dunno, maybe," I shrugged, surprised at how okay I had become with not knowing the answer.

Over the last few years, the answer has started to unfold. It has become more of a subtle way of being and living, more than any specific decision or career choice. I started my own management consultancy specializing in leadership and found that I was called to work with businesses and organizations devoted to fulfilling their mission. My clients like that I bring a strong sense of spirit into the work and encourage them to fulfill their own personal callings in work and life.

I started volunteering at our local church. No longer a practicing Catholic, I attend a rather diverse, ecumenical, non-fundamentalist Christian church right in our neighborhood. I served by helping the church support its volunteer and staff leaders. I was nominated to the Board of Trustees, and worked on the annual fundraising campaign for a few years.

I attended a leadership seminar for volunteer and ordained religious leaders, where I experienced for the first time the joy of praying with my arms up in the air; where it was okay to praise God with tears running down my face, splashing silently on the floor in front of me. I am now considering going back to graduate school, and hope to find ways to support religious and multi-cultural harmony on a global basis. All the while I have met other leaders in both my business and spiritual communities who support my deepening relationship with God.

I know I am on the right path when I hear the words that our pastor uses to close the service every week. "Go forth today and every day, living your life in such a way that others see God living in you." God is speaking to me with these words. "Hmmm," I think each time I hear it, "Live *my* life in such a way…." God's way. Kind. Open. Forgiving and steadfast. Persistent. Patient. Graceful. Thoughtful. Joyful. My call is this simple.

While out there on my journey, I have good days and bad days.

I can feel joyful about my faith, then overwhelmed about how to put it to work in the world. But thankfully, one gesture does make me laugh each Sunday. Reverend Bill's voice greets me and my family after service as we exit the church. "Sister Liz," he says, putting on a Southern drawl and speaking his evangelical roots. "Brother Bill," I reply, enjoying the irony, challenge and blessing of God's presence in my life. Who knew God had a sense of humor?

———

Elizabeth Becker (42) was born near Philadelphia and received a degree in hospitality. She worked for years in hotels and high tech and now runs a boutique management consultancy specializing in market leadership for organizations and individuals. She also writes articles on leadership and fundraises for non-profits. Elizabeth and her family live in the Bay Area where she practices yoga, sails big boats, and writes "beginner" poems. A world traveler, Elizabeth recently returned from Peru where she hiked a less-traveled route to Machu Picchu, fulfilling another lifelong call.

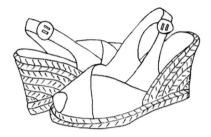

Geriatric Mama

By Lori Stott

*H*ere's the thing: I have jumped out of airplanes, scaled enormous mountains and gone diving with sharks. I have given presentations to hundreds of people, taught graduate classes at a large university and led professional board retreats.

But for the life of me, I could not figure out how to register for baby gifts.

As I lay on the soft brown couch that was quickly folding itself into my ever-growing physique, I frantically flipped through catalogs, scanned books and searched the web. This task was almost too much to bear. I worried, "How do I know which are the best products? How does anyone ever know? What if I choose the wrong ones?"

I was overwhelmed and exhausted by all of the choices. My baby was coming in two months, just after I turned the BIG 4-0. I remember thinking – perhaps due to my British-snobbery genes –

that gift registration was a rather crass practice when my husband Jay and I did it for our wedding. But, I understood. We needed stuff and people wanted to give us stuff. So why not come right out and tell them exactly what stuff we needed?

The only problem was this: I had no clue. Seriously, no clue whatsoever. I did not have nieces or nephews. Neither did Jay. Here in my adopted state of Colorado, I didn't yet have a lot of close women friends who had done the baby-thing. Or if they had, it was ten or fifteen years ago. Most of my friends were leading wilderness trips, making jewelry, writing songs and performing them, and studying the life and times of bees and beetles up at the university. They were not - most decidedly - changing diapers.

I did not know who to ask for help.

Thoughts darted through my mind: Did the baby need a crib? We planned on co-sleeping in a family bed. Did the baby need bottles? I'd be nursing. We knew she was a she so I could eliminate all the blue and green things and could concentrate on pink, purple, and yellow.

But what about a baby monitor? Did we need one with bells or lights? One that dings or dongs? Did we 'snap and go' or 'pack and play'? And what of these teeny little socks and shoes...did a newborn really need shoes?

How could baby swings and bouncy things, backpacks and blankets, Baby Einstein, baby joggers, and baby carriers possibly intimidate me? I tried to squeeze out a laugh. C'mon! I'd gone spelunking, hang-gliding, white water rafting, and rock climbing. I'd taught people who have no legs how to ski, and moved across the country solo. I had met the challenges of alcoholism (getting sober at age twenty-three), depression and infertility head-on. Why, oh why, did I break out into a cold sweat when looking at baby gear?

Ugh, the pangs of a headache were coming on.

So I rolled over, clicked on the TV and anxiously waited for my buddy. Good 'ole Dr. Phil, the one person I counted on to show up every afternoon at three o'clock. Right when I was about to pull my hair out. He was the most consistent company when I was on bed rest now for, how long was it? Twelve weeks now.

* * *

So how did I end up there? I had been blissfully pregnant. After all, it had taken two years, five surgeries (two just to correct my irregularly-shaped uterus), one birth intuitive, a Reiki master, three acupuncturists, a couple of sessions with a freaky Mayan abdominal masseuse, multiple rounds of in-vitro fertilization at two fertility clinics and finally - finally - one embryo fought its way into my uterus and decided, against just about all odds, to stay.

While my infertility issues were not necessarily caused by my "advanced" age, it did not help matters much that I was fast-approaching my fourth decade on the planet. So my pregnancy was oh-so-scrupulously monitored. And I was given two labels: "geriatric" and "high-risk."

I had actually been feeling pretty darn sprightly on the day I learned that I was a geriatric pregnant lady. I know, it just sounds wrong. My doc had been keeping a close eye on my tendency toward preeclampsia (high blood pressure, swelling, headaches). I had to have my blood drawn once a week. Walking into a new clinic, I gave my name to the woman behind the glass window. She looked at her appointment calendar and peered back up at me through her dark-rimmed glasses.

"Funny," she said with a wink, "You don't look geriatric."

"Excuse me?" I managed.

"Well, I am looking at your file from your OB's office. Says here you are a "geriatric." I suppose this means you are over thirty-eight?"

I squeaked out, "Uh huh."

What I wanted to do was shout, "Hey! I am *only* forty! Do you have *any* idea what it took for me to get here?" But I did not. I sat down in the waiting room on a hard chair and tried to lose myself in an old, tattered magazine. Ah, MORE magazine, for "women over forty." Evidence that I was not the only geriatric pregnant woman who came to this clinic.

Being called "high-risk" was indeed ironic (and sometimes even funny) given the high-risk adventures I had once embarked upon. Unlike all of those outdoor escapades, this time I was responsible for two lives, not just one.

* * *

Life is funny, ya know? It can truly change in an instant. On Sunday I was in Florida, twenty weeks pregnant, jumping up and down in the waves of the Atlantic, squealing with delight like a small child. On Monday, back in Denver in the sonogram room I was told that my "incompetent cervix" was not doing its job properly and that I would need an emergency "stitch."

When my infertility doc first informed me of this condition, I looked up the word "incompetent": inept, ineffective, "not up to it."

Another definition: "useless." Excuse me?! My cervix was certainly *not* useless, thank you very much. I had a baby growing in there, a miracle. More of a miracle than most babies! My cervix was compromised, perhaps. But not useless.

Most women discover, sadly, that they have incompetent cervixes because they miscarry. I was told that I was very lucky that my doctor had caught this, and lucky to be monitored so closely. I didn't feel so lucky at that moment, but I knew in my heart of hearts: this child was meant to come.

Lying on the cold gray table on that Monday morning, I was informed that I would need to quit working for the rest of the pregnancy. Immediately. (Me: "*What!*" Doc: "Yes." Me: "Omigod. Okay, I guess I can go over and discuss this with my boss." Doc: "*No.* There will be no driving. You will tell them over the phone." Me: "You mean I can't drive and talk to them face to face?" Doc: "That is what I mean. That is, *if* you want this baby to go to full term.")

Oh.

I asked many questions. Finally, with more than just a hint of annoyance, the doctor checked my chart again and asked me how old I was. "Aha," he grunted. Then he asked what my education level was. What does that have to do with anything? In his experience, he sighed, women with more education argue and try to negotiate such instructions, while those with less just nod and agree to these terms.

I suppose he was thankful then, that I had just a Master's degree and not a Ph.D.

The next day was April 1. Happy April Fool's Day. The procedure – an emergency cerclage – took less than twenty minutes. A MacDonald stitch. Well, at least it was a nice Scottish thing. My great-uncle in Glasgow would be proud. Essentially, my cervix was sewn up. I was told: NO sex (duh, what with the stitches and all), no hiking, walking, aerobics, or standing for long periods of time.

On Wednesday I started my new life: TWO DOWN, ONE UP, TWO DOWN. I was given strict instructions to lie on my left side (better blood flow for the baby) for exactly two hours, after which I was allowed to get up for one hour. No jump roping or salsa dancing during those precious sixty minutes, mind you. I could take a nice long shower, walk – slowly and mindfully – with my dogs, even plant a few seeds in the garden. I came to relish those hour-long respites when I could relieve my hips, my butt, my back. I began to understand why most women go through this at a much younger age. But I was happy to be pregnant, incredibly happy and grateful, too. And I knew that this was the right moment for me, and my husband; that it was happening at the perfect time in our lives.

Sometimes I went to the nearby park and sat on a large boulder by the soothing waters of the St. Vrain River. I talked to the baby girl growing inside of me and told her: listen to the water, this favorite sound of mine. I hoped she too would love water and rocks and nature.

There were moments of peace in this, by the river - a deep knowing that I was doing the right thing. There were also moments of amazement. This was probably the first time in my forty years of life that I followed the rules so strictly, so religiously. I always had a bit of the rebel in me, constantly questioning authority. I suppose as I was approaching mid-life it was indeed time to give this up, to let it go. So there I was, following the new rules, quietly and fiercely, for the life of this child. This child with whom I was already in love.

* * *

Thirty-two weeks into my pregnancy I was liberated from bed rest. I bade faithful Dr. Phil a fond farewell. (Truth be told, I never really liked Dr. Phil. I was just using him to keep me company.) I said goodbye to the labels that I had been living with: Infertile. Incompetent. Compromised. Irregular. Geriatric.

I began, instead, to think of myself as "Mommy." A mommy who had prayed, chanted, and cried; endured endless poking and prodding, operating rooms, foul-tasting Chinese medicines, injections, doctors, nurses, acupuncture needles, and blood draws; and breathed fear, endured heartache and clung to faith to bring this child into the world. A mommy who could bring her sense of adventure and love of learning to this new journey, this new life that was just beginning for me at forty.

A mommy… who had no earthly idea what type of baby monitor to get.

Lori Stott (45) lives in the foothills of the Rocky Mountains with her beloved husband and daughter, two hyperactive yellow Labradors and a cat with a mood disorder. With a Master's degree in Nonprofit Management, Lori is a professional grant writer and nonprofit consultant, and has raised money for various organizations around the county. She also does some editorial work on the side and writes essays for fun. Recently she got up on the rope swing at Open Gym Night and made "eee-eee" sounds like a monkey. She did not care that she surely looked like a total dork to the other parents, or that her body carries a little middle age around her middle. Her favorite saying: life is short.

The Naked Truth

By Elaine Hamill

Okay, so I'm not the first person to get old.

My mom got old, *her* mom got old, and some day even Hannah Montana will get old.

But it's still just as shocking and painful for me as it must have been for that first middle-aged cavewoman who pulled on her favorite saber tooth tiger-skin midriff top and found it a little snug around the bust, a little too revealing in the tummy. Lucky girl, she didn't have a mirror to confirm her fears.

Lately I've been carrying around a slow-growing panic that flashes every time I'm in a dressing room. My body is morphing into something unrecognizable. Oh sure, with clothes on, it still resembles its former self, give or take a bit of sag. But in the secret corridors of Nordstrom, Macy's, and J. Jill, it reveals itself to be an entirely new entity – something its long-time owner barely recognizes.

I view this as a complete betrayal by a collection of parts I had come to know and trust. For so long my body has lived up to my expectations – walking, standing, processing food, staying awake for daytime activities, and retrieving things that have fallen on the floor without any embarrassing noises.

But now my body seems to be lurching forward in some predestined march toward something resembling … I don't know, maybe bagged chowder. If it weren't my own, I would stare in horror the way you do at circus freaks or large mounds of elephant scat at the zoo. But it's *me* in there, and I can't believe what I'm seeing.

If this is the way the forties seem to be winding down, I'm a little worried about the next decade. I can't even look down at my legs when I walk anymore, because my knees are starting to shake with each step. Now I understand why middle-aged women in past centuries dressed the way they did – because it was okay at the time for women to assume the shape of a Mrs. Butterworth's bottle after child-bearing. Sometime since, it's been decided that we all should maintain impossibly aerobicized physiques, or risk censure from the ranks of more obsessive Boomers still able to touch their toes and wear cropped pants without looking like Miss Piggy.

I now understand why Chico's, the clothing store for ladies of a certain age, does not have mirrors in its dressing rooms. That way you never have to look at yourself naked while putting on their clothes. And when you come out to the public mirror to be fawned over by the salesclerks, you are not already in tears. Plus, you have covered your mutinous lumpiness with billows of linen, tencel and raw silk, and immediately one of the salesclerks puts a 12-pound necklace of tree bark and river stones around your neck to distract you, and you are so dazzled by your reflection that you purchase the entire outfit just so you don't have to take it off.

It's an ingenious business plan.

My husband, already in his fifties and feeling his own form of aging – which for a man consists mainly of having an aging wife – finds he has become the "old man" in his office. He works in advertising, where the age of the average worker is approximately 15. I know because I used to work in advertising, but wisely left the business at 28, already well past my expiration date. In the 1980s, frantic 20-somethings with apartments in the city and clothing budgets from Mom and Dad would happily work 80-hour weeks at ad agencies, and then spend cocaine-frenzied weekends drinking and talking about their 80-hour work weeks. I never quite fit in.

It's a hard lifestyle to maintain. If you're lucky, you get to pull out once you have kids, and then you can exchange the singles rat race for the stroller derby/soccer practice/real estate rat race. This is a period that feels like forever when it is your turn to bring snacks for the baseball team, but actually whizzes by while you are taking your youth and agility for granted.

Blink twice during your forties and the next thing you know, you're looking at your body in a dressing room mirror and – pilates or no pilates – it resembles a large cow bladder. I remember seeing Susan Sarandon, one of earth's sexiest women for a really long time, wearing jeans in *Thelma and Louise*, and thinking, "Gee, she looks like a chimp." And the last time I tried on jeans in a store? I looked like a chimp.

It sucks the fun out of reading *Glamour, Cosmopolitan,* and *Vogue*. You start to notice that you are no longer part of the magazine's target audience, because your body – through no fault of your own – no longer "responds" to the clothing or products they offer. And you can tell the magazine editors know this by the prevalence of ads for acne medication, low-riding pants that say "Juicy" across the butt, and birth control pills. You are somewhere between the daytime TV demographic for diapers and detergent, and the golden years of major network national news – the years where viewers seem to need endless rejuvenating prescription pills and intentionally vague adhesive products that promise you will be sitting on your front porch smiling some day, either because your breath is fresh, or because your husband was able to successfully do something he hadn't done for a long time

But back to the shopping. Overnight I seem to have outgrown my most favorite local high-end mall. There is nothing there for me anymore. I am too old for The Gap, too normal-sized for Banana Republic, not preppy enough for J. Crew, too cool for Talbot's, and too modest for any other place that features spaghetti-strapped dresses and stiletto heels or cork platform soles in its windows. I am even too over it to be swayed by half-price deals on mango bath salts and invigorating facial scrubbing seeds from the jungles of Goroka at The Body Shop.

At Christmas time, I went into Armani Exchange. I was older than all of the sales boys, and I weighed more than any of them too. They looked at me like maybe I would be more comfortable *not* in their store. You know, like maybe rifling through the photo drawer at Longs, or waiting for a table at Red Lobster. But I don't *feel* that old! What I feel is like the ground has shifted beneath me.

For instance, whose idea was Anthropologie? I can't imagine

a more ridiculous store. Let's see, they've got soap wrapped in parchment paper and bits of twine with French script on its label that costs $14, and odd assorted things like faucet knobs, dishtowels, and inexplicably large sea shells, all sold along with an implied Parisian lifestyle that makes no sense once you walk out the door and can't hear the Edith Piaf loop on the sound system anymore. And by the time you get over to Starbucks to order a big fat $4 American coffee, you are feeling pretty silly about the antique brass plate stand and the small flannel hand puppet you felt compelled to buy while "La Vie En Rose" was seducing you senseless.

The rest of the world might find that charming. But someone who's suddenly gotten old is immune.

I am immune to the perfume counter at the department store, which is shilling fragrances designed by actresses from MTV of whom I have never heard. I am immune to the mascara-waving 20-year-old who wants to give me "smoky eyes." I am immune to the carefully laid holiday tables and their imaginary guests who think they have just invented martinis and Cole Porter over at Pottery Barn. I am done with the charming toddler outfits that my children – now old enough to join the Coast Guard – do not need. And I am done with all of the promises sold in shopping malls, the mecca of American girls since I was, well, an American girl.

I am woman, hear me roar. But I think I'm done with the mall. Can that be possible?

My shopping bag remains empty. There is nothing out there for me anymore (unless you count the $12 jars of butterscotch sauce at Williams-Sonoma or the colored scarves at the Pashmina kiosk to cover the crepiness that has become my neck. Or maybe some drawer dividers at The Container Store.)

And this must be why old ladies stop buying clothes altogether, and instead go out to lunch, attend matinees of foreign movies and lectures at the garden club, and participate in all the other mid-life sisterhood activities America has constructed for us.

Which, even for a cavewoman, turns out to be not so terrible. We can leave those baby doll dresses and thong-baring low-rise jeans for the next generation. We're grownups, for heaven's sake.

As long as we can keep our dignity. And matching shoes and purses.

Elaine Hamill (49) teaches American Literature in a private high school in Northern California. She has been writing a bi-weekly newspaper column for eight years. She has been married to the same man for 26 years; they are almost finished raising three sons. She has taught nursery school, kindergarten, and middle school, and has worked with grown-ups in book and magazine publishing in New York City and San Francisco. She loves to cook and play the piano, and tries to avoid attending sporting events. She is still able to enjoy shopping – for shoes.

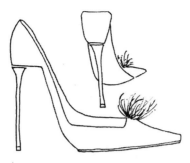

My Ambassador of Fun

By Kym Miller

"Show me a woman who doesn't feel guilt and I'll show you a man."

- Erica Jong

It started to creep in slowly, undetected, infiltrating our marriage and those once-blissful unions of our friends as well. Later I would refer to it as the "Who Had the Worst Day?" Contest. Our game started as all of life's little chores began to multiply exponentially (who knew that the co-mingling of dogs, kids, and carpets could produce so much more than the sum of their parts?), pitting my husband against me for the title of who carried more of the burden. Somewhere in the busy shuffle, we each began equating our worth as a partner with the amount of struggle endured. After a few short weeks of novice sparring, each of us stood perpetually ready to slam down the buzzer and give the more convincingly pathetic response to "How was your day?" *I had to get up at 5:00 with the kids! My meeting ran two hours late! The car stalled when I was eight miles from home! My flight was delayed for the fifth time!*

Soon, the rules of this unspoken challenge, as they had painstakingly developed, seemed to dictate that we should find new and creative ways to be burdened. Within a few months, "waiting hours for a late repair man" or "nursing a cold" had become passé and would no longer win first prize. To be truly victorious, one had to be stranded on the freeway with two flat tires, or endure a triple root canal. Heaven forbid either of us actually find delight or frivolity in our day. Running laughing through the sprinklers would have been grounds for disqualification without even a free gift bag.

Surprisingly, most of the couples around us were also engaging in similar rivalries. I remember my friend Anna calling me, so mad she could barely get the words out. "You...it's just so...you can't believe it! I got back from a four-day business trip and...it's so bad. The house is a wreck! I think all he did was play with the kids!"

"What excuse did he give?" I asked, attempting to determine who should earn more sympathy points.

"Oh, he said it was hard, really hard. Our dog threw up twice in the middle of the night. And then he gave me this pathetic look and told me he hadn't had time to do any cleaning! Like I clean the house in my leisure time!" She moaned and then recounted how every moment of her trip had been taken up with work, advance Christmas shopping and learning to pay their bills on-line. After a pause and a sigh she added, "I did get to have dinner out but I still think I had it worse."

In our marital struggle for supreme sacrifice, I'm not sure who was usually winning, but on one particularly angst-filled day I came to the disturbing conclusion that we were *both* losing. That morning found me desperately searching for the car keys while trying to herd two small children off to pre-school, only to discover that the keys were in my husband's pants pocket, hundreds of miles away. Fueled by incredulity and then a desperate wish to alter reality, I stood, repeatedly pressing the "play" button on the answering machine, listening to his deeply apologetic admission that he had moved my car before leaving for his overnight business trip, inadvertently keeping the only set of keys. "So...." His message trailed off several times, because frankly, what could he say? He ended with a weak attempt to pull himself back into the competition: "I'll probably just be eating in my room tonight so... you can call me whenever you like." Ha! Like somehow room service could possibly compete with being stranded without wheels in Toddler town. Desperate as the situation seemed, a vague notion of victory surfaced. *No way* could he top this one!

But then the strangest thoughts, perhaps borne from the fatigue of constantly subverting pleasure, began to plague my triumphant victimhood. I didn't *want* to be an irritated person all day. And what good would it do for him to be feeling so bad? Suddenly, all of this jousting seemed supremely *sub*optimal. What I actually wanted was to have fun, perhaps be a little silly, and maybe even become downright joyous. When had I let this escape from my day-to-day life? For inspiration, I had only to look at our two little girls who had chosen, during this brief respite in their mother's haste, to spin around until they were dizzy and fall laughing onto the carpet. I can still remember the rush of awareness that knocked me back to my senses.

I picked up the phone and dialed. "You know what I want?" I asked.

"What?" The hesitation in his voice making it clear that he was bracing himself for a harsh reprimand.

"I want you to be my ambassador of fun, and I want to be yours."

"What exactly does that mean?"

"I don't know – it just came to me, but I think we could help each other. Like, what are you going to do tonight, that is really enjoyable?"

"Well... they did ask us if we wanted to go to a basketball game, but..."

"I think you should!" I interrupted, "And go out to dinner too."

Warming to this amusing turn-of-events, he asked, "Well, what are you going to do today that's fun?"

"You know I think these gals and I may just take a few days off from life and goof around a little, maybe take some walks, have some ice cream, that sort of thing."

"That sounds good."

"Yeah, it does, doesn't it?"

Soon we began perfecting our new roles with written reminders like "Have a good time today" and "Don't forget to laugh" and even suggestions like "Treat yourself to a special lunch." While I rediscovered my flare for spontaneous outings, like whisking myself away for an afternoon movie, I noticed that my husband seemed to have a special guilt-free gift for incorporating more pleasure into his life without making it a grand affair. Let loose from the confines of our burdensome challenge, I would find him taking a nap on the living room couch, carpet unvacuumed, toys scattered everywhere, and the raucous tussling of our offspring filling the room. I couldn't imagine ignoring all of these demands. How was he doing it?

After much observation I realized that in terms of pure enjoyment of life, men have one key advantage: tunnel vision. Take your average female walking through her house on the way to the back deck for a few moments of rest in the sun. The sight of one rag on the counter will send her mind to the pile of undone laundry beckoning from upstairs, a pen might be a harbinger of late notices if the bills aren't paid soon, and a simple glance at the phone will remind her that it's actually been four days since her mother called. Her journey to relaxation is so fraught with subtle interceptors – not to mention all the ringing, screaming, barking kinds – that her chance of actually arriving at "down-time" fades to a blip. Take that same house, with those same booby-traps, and most men can arrive at the sacred shrine (i.e., couch, beer in hand, game on) with fewer scratches than Indiana Jones. Why? Because their eyes never left the prize. Men have the genetic predisposition to focus solely on that coveted antelope and ignore the mice scurrying at their feet. Frustrating as it may seem, I think we women have a lot to learn from this sort of rapt attention. Sure, there are occasions when that clanging alarm needs to be heeded, but mostly it seems we are reacting to a hundred little calls to attention that actually could wait a day or two, or at least an hour, while we put our feet up, have something yummy to drink, and escape into a few chapters of a favorite book.

Years after our contest came to a sudden halt, and on the eve of our twentieth wedding anniversary, our new approach has firmly taken root in our relationship. When the answering machine shows way too many unreturned messages, and the lawn needs to be mowed, my Ambassador of Fun sets the example by taking a few moments to relax before tackling the to-do list. And if he finds me leaping through hoops of obligation, he will resort to long hugs or playful words to remind me to keep it all in perspective and make time to live a little. Sometimes when we know each of our days are particularly full we like to pull each other aside and ask with a mischievous grin, "So, what are you going to do today?" While neither one of us seems destined to take home the once-coveted pity prize, this life of conspiratorial fun has finally become its own reward.

Kym Croft Miller (42) was raised in Alaska as a small shivering member of the Croft family. She eventually migrated to college in sunny Northern California to study writing and thaw out. After continuing her California hiatus by attending law school, Kym and her husband Tim moved to Portland, Oregon where they are now having a fine time with their three daughters and two Labradors. Kym is the author of several articles, as well as a juicy book proposal about the crazy year her family went without buying…anything.

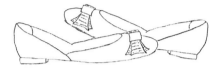

Just a Blip

By Maria Hjelm

The death of my mother defines for me a chunk of time. It's now been 24 months since she became ill, 15 months since she died, and I still reside in the era of Mom's death.

This era began on my 39th birthday, spent at the doctor's office where he told us that her suffering was terminal. Over the next nine months, I came to expect her death at any moment and even to wish for it at times, both for her sake and my own. And so I ushered in my 40th birthday with the most adult of experiences – saying goodbye.

The actual goodbye went something like this. The last few hours I had with my mother were spent watching one of the many Jane Austen film adaptations I've seen numerous times. I was secretly disappointed that she'd already viewed the Keira Knightley version of *Pride and Prejudice*, so I ran out to the closest book and video store and bought *Mansfield Park*, an artsy film that strays pretty far from Austen's book. You see, the novels of Jane Austen and their film adaptations are the most delicious candy for me. I am in awe of Austen's snappy dialogue, her brilliant characters, and her flawless story construction. And while I wouldn't bother with these books were it not for her impeccable writing, I'm a bit embarrassed to admit that I keep going back for totally different reasons. There's safety and happy endings in these books.

My mother appreciated this genre almost as much as I do. The movies and stories must have transported her. She probably read her first Austen novel when she was in high school in Sweden, and I treasure dearly her copy of *Jane Eyre* (I know, Brontë, not Austen), bound in red cloth, that she passed along to me.

On this particular day, I don't know if my Mom was transported at all. She dozed in and out of sleep, she stared at the TV screen, and she took sips of ginger ale. She was in the last weeks of life, and had been like this for many months. I was home to help and later that afternoon was to fly home to my family.

When I said goodbye to her that afternoon, I lay my face in her lap and wept. I don't think she shed a tear, as there was no liquid left in her to flow and the medication had deadened her emotions. Still, she performed her last motherly act of protection and said to me with a dismissive wave of her hand, "Forget about all this. This is just a blip."

As a parent, I too am quick to lie if I think it can prevent pain. But I knew better than to believe that this was just a blip. I still wonder, though, did she mean to protect me or reassure me? Was she already in touch with the ever-expanding universe and the eternity that was to be hers so soon? Or did she know with some certainty that we'd be together in the hereafter? Or was she referring to the fact that every child loses a parent and the circle of life elegantly negates tragedy? The ultimate entry into adulthood for me was not knowing what she meant and struggling in my own faith for guarantees that I'd see her again.

This goodbye stood in stark contrast to another one we shared while I was in college. Oddly, she was leaving me then and was moving abroad. It was not a move that thrilled her, probably because she felt deeply that it was wrong to leave her children behind, even if they were all adults. We separated from each other at an escalator. I moved to the top while she stayed at the bottom, and there was no end to the tears that flowed. In that moment, she would never have claimed that this goodbye was "just a blip."

A few weeks after our final goodbye and just a few hours before I got back to her, my Mom died. I haven't yet let go of the pain of not being with her in those last moments. I wish she had shared more with me about her feelings towards death. I watched her experience moments when she'd speak to her dead father, her dead brother – I've hoped until my heart might burst that they were there to meet her. The wondering about what she felt and how scared she was, and my worry that I'll never be with her again are now part of who I am. These traits are not invisible to my kids. They sometimes look into my eyes to assess how sad I am. And I find myself doing the same in front of the mirror, "How sad am I today?" Sometimes while driving, I do a quick assessment, "Would I prefer to stay in bed today? Wouldn't a cigarette be good right about now?"

So, here's my quarrel, my bone to pick, my beef with being 40 – it's all too adult, and I prefer to pretend that I'm still 28. You'd think that three kids, a mortgage, and a marriage that needs constant tending would have turned me into an adult, but it's the learning to live without the protection of my mother that has finally done it. Despite the chaos, the love and the joy that surround me, I feel more "on my own" than I've ever felt in my entire life.

I miss the short but reassuring phone calls that I had with her a couple of times each week.

Mom: What are you up to?

Maria: Same ol', same ol'.

Mom: Well, the weather here is beautiful, and the azaleas are in full bloom.

Maria: Hmm...my garden's a mess.

Mom: Well, I'm ordering for you a beautiful dahlia. You'll love it.

Maria: Sounds nice.

Mom: You know you're working too hard. Take it easy.

Maria: I don't know about that, Mom. I do what I gotta do.

Mom: If I were there, I'd take the kids so you could go out. Anyway, I need to go.

Maria: I love you, Mom.

Mom: I love you too.

My Dad now calls me often to tell me how much he loves me and to declare I'm doing a super job of things. But because he never stood in these mother-shoes, I've unfairly deemed him as lacking any credibility. Likewise, my husband does his best to tell me that the things I do are done well, but I just roll my eyes. More accurate and meaningful are the compliments paid to me by my kids, probably because they are so rare and never prompted.

Without the protection and approval of my Mother, I struggle to feel good about things. I've been told that 40 is often a time for women to panic about career, finances, marriage, religion. I believe that this artificial crossing of a line can throw you into a tailspin. I crossed the line, I let go of my Mom's hand, and suddenly things *are* different. I'm now one of those people who suffer from insomnia. I fret over the difficulties my children have, and I realize, matter-of-factly, that some of their problems may be my fault. Going back to work has sapped me of my confidence. I'm sorry for the many mistakes I've made in my marriage but grateful for the fact that my husband wants to keep me around.

On my 40th birthday, I dressed up in my most fabulous dress ever, shared a meal with friends that none of us had to cook, danced to my own mix of songs, and was even heard saying that "40 is the new 30." A month or two later, I had stopped making that claim, and now, because I hate to rain on any parade, I stop myself before saying out loud that 40 is in fact the new 50. I cling to the hope that this feeling won't persist. In my clearer moments, I know that I'm just an adult woman in the midst of a big change, and I refuse to believe that life stinks on this side of 40.

What I know is that grief and aging are processes; they take time. The blueness of one era dissolves slowly into the color of another. I will learn to live without my Mother, just as my children will learn to live without me. I will adjust to this feeling of being an adult, of being someone who has earned her crow's feet.

And so, on my 41st birthday, I comment to my husband that I don't actually mind getting older except for the fact that it also seems to be getting harder. In an unusual and sexy fit of wisdom, he speaks my language by quoting Carl Sandburg:

> *It is because I love you I give you for a birthday present the*
> *aurora borealis...*
>
> *When you want another aurora borealis you tell me and I*
> *will go where the aurora*
>
> *borealises grow and I will struggle and go on struggling*
> *till I lay on your doorstep, on*
>
> *your front porch, one more aurora borealis, to show I love*
> *you...*
>
> *You can see I am a struggler ready any day to struggle on*
> *to show you I love you.*

Maria Hjelm (41) has turned her professional attention towards public education after many years in the book publishing industry. She is a fund raiser for the Physics Department at a major university where she encounters topics such as neutrinos, quarks and polymers on a daily basis and delights in "dumbing them down" for the general public. Her passions are her three children and books, although the former really interfere with the latter. Maria conducts a very successful monthly author program in her hometown library and favors authors who love Jane Austen too. She'd give it all up, however, to travel with the Dave Matthews Band. Her supportive husband, Ted, has no issue with that and would happily come along.

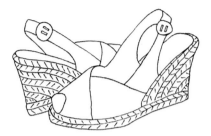

Cell Blocked

By Thea Singer

*T*he images capture my ambivalence in a heartbeat. Lying on my desk is a trio of silver-green Polaroids, each showing five to six clusters of cells, soft and grainy as Cream of Wheat and lassoed within an invisible skin. My name, identifying the clumps as mine, stares out from the labels. At one time, I thought of the snapshots, sanguinely, as baby's first pictures. They were taken from 1996 to 1998 at Cornell's Center for Reproductive Medicine and Infertility; the embryos blossomed from the union of my eggs and my husband's sperm in three in vitro fertilization (IVF) cycles.

Underneath the photos is a printout of an early home page of the Web site of the Harvard Stem Cell Institute, whose scientists announced in June 2006 that they would begin trying to clone human embryonic stem cells. The page displays four watery embryos, nearly identical to mine except that they're bathed in a pool of blue-brown light. I see these embryos as the source of possible treatments and cures for conditions ranging from juvenile diabetes to spinal-cord injuries to Parkinson's disease – no more, no less. To me, the forms are emotional light-years apart from the life-promising contours of my 16 burgeoning children-to-be.

Or are they?

Before I entered the gray world of advanced reproductive technologies (ART), in 1995, my stance was clear on what was a person and what hadn't made the leap. Embryos were not people, with a soul and a consciousness; indeed, they didn't even have body parts. They were balls of cells with the theoretical chance of growing into human beings. I was a staunch supporter of a woman's right to choose and backed embryonic stem cell research 100 percent. Friends in college had had abortions; you knew back then, even if they didn't tell you, from the boxes of thick, gauzy Kotex lying around their apartments. Choosing abortion was a difficult decision, but not an ethical dilemma.

Indeed, if you had told me before the mid-1990s that my answer to the question "When does life begin?" could become fluid, even circumstantial – based more on my psychology of the moment than on my political and religious beliefs – I would have scolded you for insulting my integrity.

I married at 40; at 41, I had a miscarriage, and the fertility doctors – alarmed at my "advanced age" – scared me straight into ART. Between the ages of 42 and 45, I went through two gamete intrafallopian transfer (GIFT) and five IVF cycles, producing 111 eggs in total, over half of which became embryos. Twenty-seven of those embryos were transferred into my body; in the GIFT cycles,

15 lone eggs were deposited into my tubes along with carefully spun samples of my husband's sperm. Even now I blanch at the numbers.

As the years progressed and the cycles failed, I slipped over some invisible cultural line. I didn't intellectually move in with the religious right. But when it came to my embryos, to my astonishment, I had emotionally set up house in their camp.

* * *

My relocation from a blue to a red state, in a manner of speaking, came hard and fast, and I followed it up with action. After my first GIFT cycle, I learned that clinics generally discard the leftover embryos they consider too lackluster to freeze. Aghast, I persuaded the embryologist for my second GIFT to freeze the extras at the one-cell stage – before they had the chance to divide and perhaps fragment – rather than assess their condition after the standard three-day wait. On the fertility clinic's consent forms, I thickly wrote my initials under the "refused" column for any requests to use my embryos for research purposes; even my eggs weren't up for grabs. I simply could not bear the thought of scientists piercing or probing or tearing them apart. The idea of selective reduction in the event of a multiple pregnancy was anathema to me, even if, I told myself, all seven embryos transferred in the third attempt (my biggest haul) were to implant.

I became uncharacteristically religious during those years – any religion, it didn't matter which – or maybe I was just in search of a talisman. I'm Jewish, but I began reciting prayers every day to Catholic saints whose pictures my husband's aunt assured me had helped make various nieces pregnant. I rubbed the belly of a friend's ceramic Buddha. And when, in 1997, we thawed my frozen embryos for transfer, I performed a ritual in the lab: hovering over the liquid-nitrogen tank where my "little ones" were banked in a test tube, I recited the Prayer for Pregnancy, in Hebrew, that my stepfather had written with a rabbi friend for me. All four embryos survived the thaw and divided (the general thaw success rate was just 50 percent), and two grew to be "perfect" six-cellers, according to the embryologist, who stood by my side during the service. We were convinced that it was the praying that got them there. Still, that IVF failed too.

Yet somewhere, through all my incantations and vetoes on consent forms, a tether to my once analytic, feet-on-the-ground self tugged incessantly. It let me know that my battle to get pregnant had more to do with control – my (until now) much-lauded ability to make things happen – than with having a child who shared my genes. Indeed, my husband and I were pursuing adoption too, with zeal, knowing the process could take time.

Now, nearly nine years later, I've drifted back over the border to my blue state. I have an eight-year-old daughter, whom we adopted at birth. True, throughout my ordeal, I remained adamantly pro-choice (for other people) and a staunch advocate of stem cell research (with other people's embryos). But it took my flesh-and-blood girl – the person who plays air flute to my air violin at Starbucks – to provide the perspective to settle my soul. I look at those Polaroids now and marvel at the transformation of sperm and egg to embryo, but I barely claim the balls of cells as mine. They are the place where, for a matter of days, my husband's and my genes met – no more, no less. Meanwhile, my baby is upstairs, waiting for me to cuddle with her in bed.

And yet... While my when-life-begins conflict has "righted"

itself, my cognitive dissonance regarding abortion has taken on a new, horrid twist: What if the 20-year-old who gave birth to my girl had made a different choice?

Just the thought stops my breath.

Thea Singer (55) has been making up for time lost in her 20s and 30s by doing what she can to have it all. A long-time features, science/health, and dance writer, her articles have appeared in numerous publications including the Washington Post magazine, O the Oprah magazine, MORE magazine, the Boston Globe, Inc. magazine, Boston magazine, Dance magazine, Natural Health, Body + Soul magazine, and the Nation. She's currently writing a book on stress and aging, to be published by Hudson Street Press. Thea lives in Brookline, Mass., with her radio-legend husband, their 10-year-old daughter and their Tibetan terrier. She hopes to write a full-fledged memoir someday, but for now remains satisfied with her six-word version of the genre: "Nature or Nurture? Strength of Will."

Essay originally published in MORE magazine, October 2006.

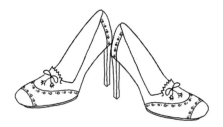

Two Writers,
One Poignant Connection

By Robin Dougherty

I am interviewing Susan Sontag when the conversation takes a sharp turn. We are speaking by phone about her new book, and then suddenly we are talking about my breast cancer.

Earlier that day my oncologist had reminded me that Sontag is also a breast cancer survivor. At first, it hadn't seemed appropriate to discuss this. It has nothing to do with her book.

So how did it come up?

Sontag was talking about the disconnect between her experience in a war zone and the lack of response from the rest of the world, the way people could watch something on TV and not take in that this horror was part of life for people just like themselves. When she'd leave the war zone and go to London or New York for a respite, people would ask her if she felt her life was in danger. What was the war like? It was as if the bombing they saw nightly on TV was taking place in another galaxy.

I see an opening. "It's startling how people, confronted with information, don't take in the reality," I say. "It reminds me of how I would tell friends I was in chemotherapy, that I had no energy, that I had been throwing up. And still, sometimes, they would not grasp that I could not go out to dinner with them."

"You had breast cancer?" Sontag asks. I can't see her, but in her voice I detect an attitude shift. She is now as avid as a scientist. She homes in on my story. "What was your diagnosis?"

We compare notes. She discovered she had a late-stage cancer in the mid 1970s, a virtual death sentence then. I was diagnosed in 2002 with metastatic disease in my back and liver. She had a double mastectomy. I had a lumpectomy. I imagine her, a young woman 30 years ago, her chest carved up, her upper arms mutilated, markedly different than the polite divot I now have in one breast, the minuscule scar near my lymph nodes.

It is astounding what people will do to stay alive, I remind myself. You never imagine you will hear your name in the same sentence as the phrase "breast surgeon." When you do, you're even more surprised to find you are willing to let a doctor cut you up.

"They told me I had a year to live," she says. No one, thank God, has given me such a grim prediction.

Sontag unleashes a battery of questions: "What drugs did you have? Where had it spread? Any recurrence?" I am markedly aware that we are no longer talking about her. I am letting go of the interview, and she is grabbing hold of it. "How old are you? How long were you in treatment?"

Like most journalists, I flatter myself that the famous authors I talk to are occasionally interested in me. It's not just prattle, I let myself believe, but an attempt to forge a connection, to make the interview more than just a businesslike interaction for an article.

At the same time, I see my journalism mentors rolling their eyes. I think of all the reporters who have made fools of themselves interviewing movie stars, rushing to light their cigarettes, imagining that the actor or actress has singled them out as special.

An interview is a make-believe conversation. I must extract the story in a limited amount of time. The author must pretend there is nothing artificial about responding to a list of questions all about her. We each have an agenda. I have a deadline. The conversation can end at any moment, when a handler pulls the famous author into another meeting. There are frequently other journalists lined up in an electronic queue, waiting to get to the author. I must use my time thoughtfully.

I glance at the clock. In one part of my mind, I am aware that I must get the interview back on track. I have five more minutes and several critical questions left to ask. The other half of my mind is thinking, "Omigod, Susan Sontag is interviewing me. She is telling me things she doesn't tell every journalist. How can I possibly interrupt?"

Thirty years ago, she explains, there weren't many options. She didn't accept the prevailing limitations. "I did some research and went to Italy." She tells me the name of her doctor, who was doing drug trials. He is now famous as a pioneer of breast cancer chemotherapy. "I underwent two years of chemotherapy, with drug X," she explains.

This is the same nasty drug that I have had, the one that makes your hair fall out, your stomach turn inside out, your immune system rebel. It is so toxic that the chemo nurses use a special kind of tubing, so the drug won't burn through the line going into your arm. I suffered through treatment for six months. She took it, in much larger doses than are given today, for two years. I think about taking drug X for two years. Two years of not knowing if it's going to work. But one year longer than her original doctor expected her to live.

"I'm cured," she says. "They won't say that but I am."

She is not the first woman I have talked to who pioneered medicine that has helped me. She is, by far, however, the longest-living survivor. I think about this.

What were the chances that Sontag, having contracted a deadly disease in 1970, might live another 30-odd years, cancer free? What are the odds that a girl who was 11 in 1970 would later cross the path of the woman who participated in trials for a drug that would save the girl's life, too? Why is there no word for this circularity of experience that unites the two of us?

I take charge again, but not before Sontag tells me I can call her to talk anytime. She doesn't mean about her work. We are connected by something much bigger than journalism. I have her number and she has mine.

Robin Dougherty died of complications from breast cancer on May, 21, 2005, at age 45. During her much-too-short career, she wrote incisive essays, features, and theater and TV criticism – as a staff writer or freelancer – for numerous publications, including the *Boston Phoenix, Washington Post, Salon, Entertainment Weekly, Miami Herald,* and *Miami New Times.* From 2001 until the week she died, she wrote the *Boston Globe*'s literary-interview column, delivering keen insight into the work of authors ranging from David Halberstam and Michael Chabon to Caroline Kennedy and Steven Pinker.

The essay above originally appeared in the *Boston Globe* on June 12, 2005. Robin wrote it after an interview with Susan Sontag, who herself died of complications of acute myelogenous leukemia in December 2004. This essay reprinted with permission of the Dougherty Family.

Thea Singer writes:

"Robin and I were friends for more than 20 years – through my 40s and well into hers. She gave me the hormone shots for my IVFs in the early mornings, when my husband wasn't around – she became expert by inoculating an orange (see my essay, *Cell Blocked*). Robin had the uncanny gift – among many, many others – of helping you believe in yourself even when every inch of you told you not to. She was so smart and funny and loving that you trusted her instincts more than your own.

I miss her immeasurably."

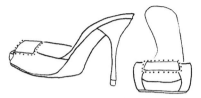

Diary of a Modern Spinster

By Anita Drieseberg

I'm a proud 42-year-old spinster. A swinging single. Career gal. No kids. I love being single. I love the freedom. I love having a sink full of dirty dishes and no one there to judge me for it. I only have to do my *own* laundry. And NO YELLING. There is never any yelling. A nice thing about being a spinster is that you can have a bunch of stuffed animals on your bed without seeming like a sexual predator. So that's a plus.

Like most women of my generation and older, I was taught that I'd get married and have kids, whether I liked it or not. It was just a fact of life. You are going to get your period, and you are going be a wife and mother. End of story. No one told me that I'd have to search for a husband or struggle to have a child. They were just going to show up and I was going to have to deal with it. The funny thing is, I don't know where I got this information. My parents married relatively late in life, and ended up infertile, eventually having to adopt. My mother was 40 when she brought me home – and that was back in 1966. Becoming a wife and mother certainly didn't fall into her lap. Yet, despite this knowledge, I still believed my destiny was preordained.

Our generation was also taught that we were going to have a career, which was cool with me. When I was a kid, I never fantasized about proposals or weddings. That wasn't glamorous, that was just a fact of life. Instead, I'd fantasize about my future career: Actress, Chef, Window Dresser, whatever. But then I'd have to give myself the reality check: Oh yeah, somewhere in there I've got to fit in the husband and the kids. Ugh. Even in my fantasies I was going to be strapped for time.

So I grew up, and over the years I've had my share of lovely and not-so-lovely boyfriends, but few were marriage material – in fact almost none of them are married to this day. I used to think it was my bad luck that I hadn't found a husband, but by 40, I had to admit that I was unconsciously choosing certain types of men. Artists, musicians – bohemian-types like myself. Eventually I realized that whenever I met a marriage-minded man, I would always hightail it out of there. What a revelation! I knew that I "created my own destiny" when it came to my career, but it took a long time before I took the same responsibility for my romantic life.

In my early 30s I went to a psychic. When I asked him if I was ever going to get married and have kids, he said, "If you wanted to have that, you would." I thought: *What a quack!* As if I have a choice in the matter. But now I know he was right. When I want something, I find a way to get it. I never knew for sure if I *wanted* the marriage and the kids. The fact that I don't have them tells me that I never really wanted them. But I'm not kidding myself, if all my friends were married, or I lived in a suburb surrounded by families, I'd feel the pressure. I'd feel there was something wrong with me. But I'm an artist in San Francisco. Half my friends are gay. The others are mostly single too. The few who married and had babies have mostly dropped off the radar. It's a different world than my mother and her generation knew.

Obviously this whole issue has been on my mind for most of my life, but it was upon turning 40 that I really confronted it. These days the number means a lot less than it used to, but there's one thing that it does still symbolize: pregnancy is probably out of the picture. I know, plenty of women have kids in their 40s, but plenty more try and can't. And those who do often have complications and birth defects. Yadda yadda yadda. Suffice it to say, I no longer see it as a possibility for me – and wow, how liberating *that* has been! No more feeling that weird combination of guilt and dread when I see babies. Now I just think: "Awe, cute!" and move along. In fact, if anything, I also think "That poor woman!" Because, after living alone for so long, I've become very lazy and selfish, and those are two things you can't be with a baby in tow. Although I have to admit I do feel some envy when I hear of male friends having kids. I think how much more into it I'd have been if I were a man. They get to have the kids without the pregnancy, the labor, the breast feeding and, most disturbing to me, the career compromise. I'm never envious of Moms, I admire them and feel for them. But Dads? Yep. Kind of jealous.

At 38 I went through a horrible break-up. Made worse by the fact that I was so close to 40. I thought he was "The One." I had thought then that maybe I would get married after all, and maybe even have a kid. When it ended, I felt like I'd lost my last chance. It was one of the hardest times of my life. I'm not getting any prettier or thinner, and it had taken me 36 years to find that guy. What were the chances of finding another? To have a 40th birthday with no boyfriend, much less no husband, was rough. My official position was that I was living the glamorous life of a career gal in fabulous San Francisco. It got me through the day. Later I found out that, though it's hard to *turn* 40, it's really not hard to *be* 40. In fact it's pretty fun!

I make a very good living working at home as a computer animator. Often I stay up all night working and sleep all day. Sometimes I take a day off, just because I can. I have a fine art studio, and am planning a show in the fall. I'm finishing up my short film, and working on a new online series. These things are my priorities. Then there's the swimming and hula-hooping (yes hula-hooping, don't knock it until you've tried it!). Add in a fairly active social life and, well, you get the picture. There aren't enough hours in the day to get everything done. They say that after a certain age, women are less likely to get married, not because they can't, but because they are so comfortable in their lifestyle that they don't want to give it up. That's me in a nutshell.

Yes, there is still the matter of the "status" that having a man affords a woman, especially among other women. "Single" still means you are lacking, no matter how full your life might be. On bad days it does affect me. But most of the time I am genuinely thrilled with this little independent life I've built for myself. I'm liberated from the fairytale now, and it has been empowering. I've realized something about myself that I think others knew all along: my purpose is to be creative. I was given special talents and those are the focus of my life. I wasn't cut out to be a superwoman. Some women can do it all: Wife, Mother, Career Woman and Artist. Not me. Something would have to suffer. Even now, there are days I can barely get around to feeding myself! Half the time, my apartment looks like a bomb hit it. Luckily, I have enough disposable income to order in food and have a cleaning lady sort through the rubble.

I've only been doing this 40s thing for two years, but so far I have to say, I'm really enjoying it. I'm basically living the same type of life as I was ten years ago, except with more money, more freedom, and less concern about the size of my butt. Empirically, I am probably "uglier" than I've ever been, but I feel more attractive than ever. I can't explain why. Maybe it's because no one expects a 42-year-old to look like a supermodel. Even supermodels don't look like supermodels once they are in their forties. The pressure's off. I started doing stand-up comedy about six months ago - something I never would have had the courage to do at 30. I was too self-conscious. Too afraid of failure or of looking like a fool. Now, I just don't give a crap. Looking stupid is a risk I am willing to take, and I highly recommend it.

So what comes next? I have so many plans for my career: my art, my films, my comedy. I can't wait to see what's waiting around the corner. Maybe I'll meet a man after all. Maybe a divorcé with kids of his own. Or maybe I'll be single forever, and I am just fine with that. Does that make me a weirdo? Probably. Does being a weirdo make me a better artist? I think so. Are there moments of self doubt and wishing I was more "normal?" Yeah, but fewer and fewer as I get older. I'm happy with the way things have turned out. I like being 42. Although now I seem to be growing a beard. Frankly, *that* I could live without.

———————————

Anita Drieseberg (42) is an Animator/Illustrator/Artist/Comic. Originally from Toronto, Canada, she has lived by herself in a small apartment in the gayest of gay neighborhoods in San Francisco since 1996. She is not gay. She is a Spinster. She likes the word Spinster and thinks all Spinsters, male and female, should embrace the word and infuse it with positive energy, and all the wonderful things the word represents: freedom, independence, and complete and utter control over the television remote.

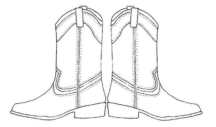

My Parents are Golden.
My Brother and I Are More Like Recycled Tin Foil. And That's On a Good Day.

By Mardi Link

*R*ecently, my parents celebrated their 50th wedding anniversary. To mark the day, they invited a hundred friends and family members to cruise Michigan's Saginaw Bay in an open-air tour boat, and then head over to their church for a chicken dinner. The event was fitting for two active people in their seventies who have an ideal marriage, are ideal parents, and who have achieved their vision of the American Dream. Together, they have good health, financial security, a propensity toward good deeds, and, no kidding, good looks.

While I watched the two of them stand united on the gangplank and greet the odd assortment of guests – their sailing friends, our frail Aunt Eunice, their Lutheran pastor and his wife, the cousin with the leftist political T-shirt – I wondered what happened to my brother and me. With parents like these, how could we have gone so wrong? Between us we have three marriages (one common-law), two divorces, two DUIs, five kids, a propensity toward beer and/or vodka and/or marijuana, two bad credit ratings, and a history of disconnected telephones. What the hell?

I asked my brother about this when I went to the tiny old trailer park where he lives with his guns and his new girlfriend. I was there to pick them up – he and his girlfriend, not the guns – and give them a ride to the anniversary party because neither has a valid driver's license. In a random attack of bad luck, within the past week each of them had been stopped by a small town cop, each had been ticketed for driving with an expired license, and each had their expired license re-taken away. Under the threat of jail now, they weren't driving. When I got out of my mini-van at the trailer park, an old man without shoes or a shirt pointed at me and yelled, "Hey! She ain't from in here!" Must have been the new skirt from Talbots that alarmed him. Black, with little pink flowers. I flip him off. "Just because I don't live here, buddy, doesn't mean I don't belong." He sat back down in his broken lawn chair, appeased.

"Not everyone can be like them," my brother tells me, once I'm safely inside the bosom of his doublewide. "Not everyone wants to be." For the first time, it occurs to me that he's okay with this. He's okay with the continental drift of difference between our parents' lifestyle and his own. I, on the other hand, am not.

I want the suburban house so clean that a Mop-n-Glow commercial could be filmed there. I want the lawn that no dandelion would dare deface. I want the garage with the organized shelves and the neatly bundled newspapers and the lawn mower that will start on the first pull because it just had an oil change. I want the marriage that is solid gold.

Logically, I know that in order to have these things, I would first have to give up the vodka, the impulse buying, the fun I had bartending, the two incontinent dogs, the two even more incontinent cats, the old farmhouse, the three unruly sons and, gulp, the boyfriend with the Harley-Davidson. I don't care. The day before the party, I walk into my parents' house after a three-hour drive, and there are no weird smells, no grit or pet hair on the floor, no dishes in the sink, no food wrappers on the counter, no strife of any kind, and I want it.

Hugs all around. "How was the traffic?" my father asks, setting aside the newspaper. "Aren't you glad you have the van? It's so good on gas. What are they getting for a gallon up north?" And then my mother: "Are you boys hungry?" she asks my sons. Behind her is a fully set table, ice in the water glasses, and matching dishes heaped with steaming homemade food. There are placemats. There are candles. There are special occasion napkins. "Your hair looks cute," she says to me. I wonder if my kids wish we lived like this. I wonder if we lived like this when my brother and I were little, or if my parents have perfected this art of gracious ease only in their later years. Thinking back to when I was a girl, I don't remember our house ever being dirty. I don't remember our telephone ever being shut off. I don't remember ever climbing into the backseat of a car that wasn't freshly washed, with a basket of snacks and a bag of my favorite toys inside.

My own family life, especially now that I'm a single parent, is lived with a slightly different, um, shall we say, "tone" than the one that permeated my own childhood. I work full time, so during summer vacations, my three sons participate in a crazy quilt of loosely-timed activities that give them some degree of supervision, without costing too much. These activities range from rock band practice with the neighborhood ne'er-do-wells in our garage, to soccer clinics that offer scholarships on a "no questions asked" basis, to church daycamp with the Congregationalists. "Where are the damn Bibles!" I remember yelling one morning when we were late. Again. In between these activities, at home supervising themselves, the three of them have become quite accomplished at video games. Let me tell you, it's a proud moment when you take your boys to the mall for some early back-to-school shopping, make a detour into the arcade, and within minutes your youngest is dwarfed by a crowd of pale, greasy teens transfixed by this little guy's prowess at Tekkan 3. A proud, proud moment. Though not exactly something you'd share with the grandparents.

At the party, the strain of parenting alone begins to show. All three boys have been asked by my parents to act as waiters, circulating amongst the guests with platters of cheese, crackers, and fruit. I overhear my 16-year-old bashing President Bush to my grandfather, whose monetary contributions to the Republican Party are legendary. The middle kid is throwing random items over the side of the boat: ice cubes, a grape, a pacifier, cheese slices, in a rapid-fire re-creation of David Letterman's gag, "Will It Float?" My father has taken a makeshift tip cup away from my youngest, but not before it has been stuffed with dollar bills. I make a silent pact with myself to transform into Attila the Mother on the ride home tomorrow.

That night, the boys and I sleep at my parents' house, under sheets that smell like lavender. The next morning, my father says he is headed back to the church where we had dinner after the cruise. "Why?" I ask. "Did you forget something?" No, he says, he needs to pick up his lawnmower. Before the party he had noticed that the church volunteers hadn't mowed the courtyard lawn, and he wanted the place to look nice for the dinner, so he mowed it himself. His Toro was still there.

"And when I get back, you need to take me over to the State Park to get the motor home. I have to drive it over to the mechanic." The motor home had been parked lakeside, at a nearby campground, and relatives visiting for the celebration had stayed in it. The refrigerator had leaked coolant for some undetermined reason and the whole thing now reeked of ammonia. My father had already gone on the Internet and was perturbed to find out that it will cost $1,200 to fix.

"While you're out, stop at the pharmacy and pick up my cholesterol pills," my mother tells my father. "And get me some Zinc. I think I'm coming down with something. Probably all the stress."

What is this? Broken things? Tasks left undone? Sickness? Unforeseen expenses? Could it be . . . dandelions on this perfect retirement lawn?

A memory comes into my head then, unbidden. I am eleven years old and just home from school. My stay-at-home mother has gone back to work as an elementary school teacher, and at the end of the day, my brother and I get home an hour and a half before she does. My father, a school administrator, will be home hours after that. There are partially unpacked moving boxes everywhere and no furniture in the family room. My brother sits on the floor, cross-legged in front of a black and white TV. This is the biggest house we've ever lived in, and it will be months before my parents can afford to fully furnish it.

I am hungry, and decide to make myself a peanut butter and jelly sandwich. There is no bread cut, so I find a freshly baked loaf my mother must have stayed up late the night before to bake, and start cutting. I hack through three-quarters of it and still don't have two slices of bread. My mother comes home right then, sees the pile of crumbs, and immediately begins to cry. I must have felt surprise and shock at her reaction. After all, to my eleven-year-old self, it was just a loaf of bread. But now, remembering, I can feel her helplessness. It wasn't just bread, it was a longing for some small sense of perfection that would not come. It was the futility of even trying to achieve it. Of trying to work full time, and still bake homemade bread, keep the house in order, the lawn mowed, and the children watched over and fed.

I want to go back in time and tell her that even approaching that kind of perfection will take fifty years to accomplish. But she knows this now, and so does my father. My brother knew it all along, or, perhaps, doesn't really care. So I tell myself instead. And, when the kids and I get home, I'm going to bake some homemade bread. I've got a really great recipe from my mom.

Mardi Link (46) is a writer and single mother of three teenaged sons. She lives in Northern Michigan on a little farm she calls The Big Valley, in deference to Victoria Barkley, aka Barbara Stanwyk, who starred in the television show of the same name. Much to her parents' pride and chagrin, Mardi divorced her husband of 18 years and has worked as a police reporter, bartender, street tree planter, tournament pool player, and seamstress. Being a writer seems tame to them in comparison, but is really the most exciting job choice of all.

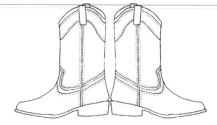

Strung Together

By Ana Ammann

I loved rock and roll. While my friends were still playing with their dolls, I was playing with my AM transistor radio; pen and paper in hand deciphering the lyrics from my favorite songs. I was obsessed with music. Each week I couldn't wait until Saturday to hear which song reigned #1 on Casey Kasem's American Top 40.

The relationship with my Fender started out innocently enough. I first saw him when my family and I were walking by our small, local music store. I peered in the windows and caught sight of a magnificent, sparkly, cobalt blue electric guitar - I could not take my eyes off him. Dad suggested we go in and look around. I was smitten and remember wanting it more than I wanted anything. Since my Dad wasn't the kind of guy to spoil his kids (if you wanted something, you had to earn it), we made a deal. He agreed to buy me that shiny blue Fender if I completed a year's worth of classical guitar lessons. A year sounded like an eternity, but it seemed worth it.

For twelve months I studied classical guitar with Mr. Rodriguez. Learning scales and how to read music was tedious – not to mention tough on the fingertips. But I figured it would be worth the pain to be able to finally hold Electric Blue in my hands and play.

A year later there he was, hanging high up on a wall, with *Fender* scripted across his head, patiently waiting for me to take him home. "Hello, Blue," I whispered as the clerk handed me the guitar, "Ready to go home?" Surprised that he was so heavy, I nearly dropped the guitar. I threw the strap over my neck and, unable to bear his weight, stood hunched and awkward. The grace and poise I had envisioned eluded me.

I looked over at my father and saw doubt and uncertainty in his eyes. Without the slightest understanding of what he was about to do to me, he said, "You can't even carry it. Too bad, it's just too heavy for you."

I couldn't believe my ears. So what if I couldn't carry it? Hadn't I earned it? "I could play it sitting down," I protested, but as I attempted to play seated, the glossy-blue back betrayed me and slipped off my leg, slipping away from me. And then it was gone.

We left. I wanted to yell after my dad about the unfairness of it all and tell him I was angry he broke his promise, but the words just weren't there. I was scared to stand up to him. I was a pleaser. A sweet little girl who never talked back, avoided conflict, and had a deep-seated need to make others happy.

I felt the tears burning in my eyes and my throat starting to close. As I hid the tears streaming down my face, I decided right then and there that I was done with the guitar.

My dad and I never spoke of that day, but as my first real disappointment, it left more than an impression. I carried the feelings around like a backpack that I refused to put down, getting heavier every time someone disappointed me. To this day my father has no idea what a profound effect his broken promise had on me. He doesn't know because I never told him.

Eventually, I traded in my acoustic strings for tennis strings. Tennis led to college, and college to a career. I had chosen the safe path, following the life plan that was expected of me. I achieved everything I set out to do and excelled. I should have been proud, but the rocker girl within me was struggling to get out.

During the work day, I was *Ana the Businesswoman* - showing up at the office in my Ann Taylor double-breasted suits, Coach briefcase, leather pumps, tasteful makeup, and conservative hair. Days were spent in meetings with company executives and lunch with other young, upwardly mobile leaders.

But at the end of the day, I transformed into a completely different person. Sporting dark, punky spikes with burgundy streaks (that would wash out in my morning shower), dark shadows on heavy, black-rimmed eyes and Doc Martens, *Ana the Rocker Girl* would hit the clubs, mingle with the fray and listen to alternative rock bands. Bright red lipstick contrasted starkly with my pale white skin and shiny black leather motorcycle jacket. I would move through the thumping, over-crowded clubs like an undercover agent, hoping that my daytime identity would not be discovered.

When I became a wife at 27 and a mother at 29, the compartmentalization of my personas became even more complicated as I tried to balance who I was to my employer, my husband, my family, my friends and my son. I felt as though I was adapting to my environments like a chameleon, yet none of those environments were entirely mine. I no longer had a place in the world that belonged to just me, and I was not fully present in any of the roles I was playing.

By the time I was 33, I didn't know who I was anymore. As I say that, I am painfully aware of just how overused and new-agey that statement sounds, but it was my reality. The pleaser I had been as a little girl carried over into my adult life and I became everything that everyone else wanted me to be and nothing for myself. I had mastered career and motherhood, but had grown disrespected and disregarded in my marriage. I could no longer breathe being defined by what my husband expected, what I did for a living, the neighborhood I lived in, or the circles I traveled in.

So I wiped the slate clean, got a divorce, moved, and started over. In this new situation, I had no reputation to live up to or expectations to meet. It was all up to me. Thankfully, I still had my career and my amazing little boy, Henry, who was the center of my universe. I was petrified and exhilarated.

And then one day, I found what I'd been looking for. It was in the local newspaper: "Volunteers Needed for First Ever Rock & Roll Camp for Girls." Without a moment's hesitation, I picked up the phone and dialed. "Hi," I said to the timid girl who answered the phone, "I'm calling about the ad in the Mercury seeking volunteers. Can I please speak to the Camp Director?"

"I am the Camp Director," the plaintive voice replied, "and I'm so overwhelmed, I don't know what to do."

In the end, I saved her. And she saved me. For the first time in my life, I was able to meld both my Rocker Girl and Business Woman personas. It was empowering and fulfilling.

What had started out as one woman's class project to teach 20 girls music for a week, turned into a girl's rock revolution based in Portland, Oregon. Word of the camp spread fast and far. Within a week we had received more than 250 applications from as far away as Boston.

The girls with greatest need were given priority. Tara, a 12 year-old self-described outsider, had spent the past three years in foster care while her mother worked to overcome drug addiction. In her application essay, she wrote about having to move around, never fitting in with her foster families or schools, yet being grateful for her guitar which she considered her best friend. Tara desperately wanted to meet other girls like her who would accept her.

The week before camp was set to start, we found out that Tara's mother sold all their possessions – including Tara's guitar – to pay for a fix.

The news was devastating to me. Camp wouldn't be the same for Tara without her guitar.

I couldn't stand to think that Tara was going to miss out on the one bright thing in her life because of her mother's mistake. I remembered how crushed I felt that day in the guitar store and just couldn't let this girl's dream die as mine had.

I got in my car and drove to the nearest Guitar Center, walked in and pointed to a sassy-looking red Fender Bullet on the wall.

"Wrap it up!" As I spoke, I wondered why I had never done that for myself? But even though the guitar wasn't for me, finally buying the Fender healed me. It had taken more than 30 years, but the camp and the girls finally brought music into my life.

I'm 40 now, no longer that little girl who waited to be told what she could and couldn't do. Rather than allow my surroundings to define me, I define myself. Instead of thinking about what is expected of me as a daughter, friend, employee, partner or mother; I think about what I expect – better yet, what I *want* – for myself and go after it with the confidence that music gave me.

After years of struggling to keep my different identities (that ranged from June Cleaver to Joan Jett) apart, I now embrace all of them every day. I love being a devoted mother who can work all day, make it to the baseball game in time to see Henry pitch a no-hitter, plan a year of projects to support women in music, score tickets to see a Depeche Mode concert with my best friend, strum a few bars of a favorite song on my guitar and bake a mean batch of oatmeal cookies before calling it a day.

I am now the proud owner of five guitars, and my favorite is a sparkly, cobalt blue electric Fender.

Ana Ammann (40) is a business consultant, published music journalist and advocate of women in the arts. She coordinates Portland's "Support Women Artists Now" (SWAN) Day celebration, and contributes to the leadership of the Siren Nation Festival, Portland Women's Film Festival (POW Fest) and ROCKRGRL Music

Conferences. She is working on her first book about British post-punk bands from the '80s and is starting a foundation called *Girls & Guitars* to provide free guitars, music instruction and mentorship to girls in underserved communities between the ages of 10 and 15 across the country.

The View from a Broad

By Therese Gilardi

*I*t's taken me decades to drag myself into an athletic club. And I would have happily avoided the gym forever, since a room full of exercise equipment is about as appealing to me as an organ transplant, but for the fact that the local Club Med is the only place with decent water pressure in my Paris neighborhood. Granted, most women join an expensive gym with a fitness, rather than hygiene, regimen in mind; however, I was confident it was money well spent as I made my inaugural visit to the Club. I breezed past the exercise machines, with nary a glance, and pushed through the gray metal locker room door into a fest of human flesh.

Everywhere I turned there were women: tall women, short women, black women, white women, young women, old women, gay women, and straight women, all with one thing in common – their complete lack of clothing. These Parisian women sashayed through the aisles, lounged on the benches, and admired themselves in the far-too-clean mirrors, their Club towels carelessly next to or under, but never around, them. I had not seen such a spectacle since the winter my then four-year-old daughter had taken to lolling about in the nude in front of the space heater. (What can I say? She was one when we moved to France; she has a European sensibility.)

Now, my first instinct was, of course, to flee. I was certain that not even the most hard core of pornography films featured anyone in the positions some of these reclining women had assumed. But if I left, then I would have missed my shower, and spent those hundreds of euros of membership fees in vain. So I looked down at my feet and shuffled toward a free locker. Slowly people began calling out "bonjour," so I was forced to look up. Once I did, I couldn't tear my eyes away.

All around were captivating new sights, but none so outrageous as the ways these women had chosen to groom their "private" hair. I felt like I had a front row seat at a rather unconventional fashion show, where all of the models sported their own signature "looks," as distinctive as the couture shops that line Avenue Montaigne. One young woman had little Salvadore Dali mustaches lying against her otherwise hairless torso. Another had a small blue jewel at the top left corner of her pubic bone, twinkling against what looked like a pre-adolescent's body. Several older women had variations of the French "bob": a conservative, fairly short hair-do with uniform length all around. Although the designs varied, every one of them had pubic hairs that were as sculpted and trimmed as the gardens of Versailles.

Despite having given birth twice, I had never discussed, let alone seen, any attention paid to this area of the body before. I grew up in a time and place where such body parts were never mentioned, let alone adorned. I am still not entirely convinced that a "Brazilian wax" is not some sort of remedy to be slathered against the side of one's car. I was shocked, to say the least, as I tentatively glanced up at the other women in the locker room, hoping they would not think me some sort of unkempt slob, but, rather, the caretaker of a body that resembled a wild, slightly neglected and overgrown English garden.

I needn't have worried. For, while I, the good forty-something American, tried to fold into myself (as I had years ago in gym class) the women around me had no such qualms. They gestured while speaking to me, oblivious to my discomfort, since, to them, walking around and chatting *au naturel* was as normal as breathing. Indeed, they were as thrilled with their bodies as an infant is when he discovers his hands. No matter what her age or body type, each woman appeared comfortable with herself, holding herself erect in a proud manner I am certain I have not adopted since the age of two.

I finished my shower as quickly as possible and fled, fairly disconcerted by what I had seen, although I couldn't put my finger on why. I've lived in this country three separate times since the age of twenty; I know that the French use topless women to sell everything from oven cleaner to children's yogurt. They are so comfortable with visions of female nudity that they have adopted the bare-breasted Marianne, whose image graces many public buildings, as the symbol of the republic. Still, though, I was ill at ease; it took me a full ten days before I made it back to the Club, half wondering if the unconventional scene I'd witnessed was some sort of exception. Perhaps there had been a group of nudists in the shower last time.

The new bathers who greeted me on my second visit were the

same as the women I encounter on the beach in France, where my daughter and I are often the only females not taking "the girls" out for some fun in the sun. Once again, these Gallic women were completely unselfconscious, admiring themselves, gently caressing their bodies, and meowing like cats while they relaxed in the sauna.

As I watched them, that sense of discomfort I had felt days earlier returned, morphing into a tidal wave of immense grief that the women of my culture never feel so at home in their own bodies. I thought about the myriad ways American women are taught to feel ashamed or even afraid of their bodies, from the "offensive odors" we are supposed to associate with menstruation, to the heavy-handed, overly frightening advertisements and stories that pepper our airwaves. Add to that noxious cocktail the far-too-prevalent notion in our youth-obsessed culture that women over forty are no longer as physically or sexually alluring, and it's no wonder so many of us are reaching for the Botox.

I can't help wondering, though, if there isn't some correlation between artificially enhancing our bodies and a lack of familiarity with them. I know that, after several months at Club Med, I became so comfortable walking around in the buff that my inhibitions eventually evaporated like the steam in the hammam. One day, on a trip to England, I even found myself automatically stripping down in the poolside sauna, much to the horror of my fellow bathers.

I don't know for sure if there are locker rooms like the one at Club Med across the Atlantic – places where women lounge and interact with each other in the nude, but if there are, I'm willing to bet that they are an anomaly. We Americans have no frame of reference of the unclothed female form as an object of beauty, or even just as a being. Most of us have no experience of communal nudity. I would venture to guess that the majority of American women are like me; I have never seen any of my female family members, with the exception of my daughter, unclothed. We are a country where nursing mothers are shunted off to private rooms lest the sight of a breast or, God forbid, a naked nipple, offend someone, where we hide the lower half of our body from our own vision at the doctor's office. By contrast, if a French woman were handed a sheet by a physician, she would assume it was something to sit on. We have no art or tradition that celebrates nudity, not even knowledge of the fact that, for many women around the world, the communal bath is a source of pleasure and companionship.

Why does this matter? Because, although we are so much more than just our bodies, there is no denying the fact that they are, at least in this lifetime, an integral part of our being. In order to feel as powerful as we should, we need to love and cherish our bodies to earn respect and admiration for them, no matter what their shape or size. And that is very hard for any American woman to do, especially for those who are dismissively called "of a certain age."

It's only now that I am on the fun side of forty that I recognize where the great divide lies between my native culture and my adopted homeland. In American culture, I see it in the absence of over-forty women appearing on the silver screen, in the lack of older women featured in magazines that my husband brings back from the US, and in the deluge of television ads that tell us that we are somehow not all right just the way we are.

In all honesty, I probably wouldn't have noticed this ageism to the extent that I have, if not for the daily encounters with billboards featuring European actresses and public figures, complete with lined faces and yellowing teeth. Am I saying French culture is somehow superior, that the French are, as they themselves would no doubt attest, the only true connoisseurs of living? Not on your life. The longer I live in Europe, the more entrenched I become in my pride at being an American; we are, after all, the best people on the planet at reinventing ourselves, the ones that the rest of the world looks to in ways I never even imagined until I moved abroad.

But, you see, we have this little glitch when it comes to viewing, accepting and loving the beautiful variety of bodies in our over-forty female population. It seems to be one of the few areas in which, eternal optimists that we are, Americans focus on the glass being half-empty. I know from whence I speak; my body bears the scars of operations, childbirth, miscarriage, and years of hard living, marks I am far too prone to focus on, a habit regularly reinforced by all of those women's magazines that, while claiming to feature the "mature woman" (God, I hate that phrase, don't you?), really serve as sales vehicles for peddlers wishing to sell the elixir of youth.

My years in France, though, have taught me that I have been looking at things from the wrong perspective. I need to see my body the way a French woman sees hers: as a secret garden to be cultivated (and groomed) simply because it is mine. Now make no mistake; this is a country enamored of plastic surgery. But the difference is that the women here strive to be better versions of themselves, at their current age, rather than shadowy reproductions of the girls they once were.

I'm in the process of moving to Los Angeles, a city not known for its infatuation with the over-forty woman. I'm not worried, though - the first thing I packed was the lesson I learned at Club

110

Med: that my body is special and beautiful just because it's mine. My new house has a beautiful bathroom, complete with powerful shower. I know I'll enjoy it, although I suspect that such solitary grooming will not be nearly as rewarding as the communal bathing experience I've come to love.

Therese Gilardi is a writer whose work has appeared in literary and parenting magazines, as well as in the book "So Far And Yet So Near: Stories of Americans Abroad" and the upcoming "Hungry Paris." She lives with her husband, two children, and assorted pets. When she's not writing, Therese can be found hanging out in the locker room at Club Med.

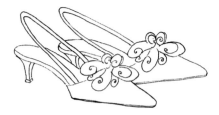

On Being Single

By Samantha Pinney

I was trying to get dressed for work. Clothes were strewn about the room though I kept reaching deep into the back of my closet for more. Wrong fit, wrong color, wrong look. Tears welled up in the corners of my eyes as my emotions crept to the surface. I sat down on the edge of the bed and took a few deep breaths trying to collect myself. Relax. Focus. Exhale. I stood up and pulled a wrinkled outfit together from the floor, grabbed my sunglasses and purse, took one last look in the mirror, and burst into tears.

It wasn't always like this. Relationships came and went. Some stayed with me more than others after they ended. One left me devastated for more than a year. But until recently it never occurred to me that there might not be a *next* relationship when the last one came to its conclusion. Even during the dry spells – over months, over years – I still felt optimistic, never mind stumbling through drunken flirtations and depressing dates. I still had hope despite the tidal waves of emotion that bowled me over me from time to time.

There was the egotistical, but geographically desirable and wittily sarcastic, Dave. We liked the same articles in the New Yorker, listened to the same music, had the same taste in food, movies, and men's cologne. We dated with the understanding that it was casual. No strings attached. I googled "casual sex." Articles and testimonies suggested that casual relationships rarely ended well, but he filled a void in my life – physically and mentally. I briefly considered the outcomes and decided that I was empowered, not compromised. I was there by choice, not necessity. At least, that was my mantra. Naturally, things didn't end well – not because either of us got more attached but because one day he just didn't return my call, and I never heard from him again. I know he's still in San Francisco. A question mark dotting the Bay Area landscape, another part of my past I catch myself thinking about from time to time. In my delusional moments, I imagine that he has a girlfriend or wife, maybe a child, a big golden retriever, a house in Tahoe or on the coast where he invites friends for the weekend. And I have to wonder – did I miss the obvious? Could it all have been mine for the taking? Does everyone fantasize that their ex's have gone on to lead far superior lives than when they were with you?

Fortunately, common sense and anti-depressants save me from myself when doubts about my past decisions arise. And a hundred different quotes about fate, circumstance and the unknown. And my girlfriends, who insist he was always a loser. God, I love them. But increasingly, as I get older, each failed relationship takes a little more out of me, and my resilience diminishes ever so slightly.

I wanted desperately to love Andy, the sexy, kind-hearted, motorcycle-riding smoker who seemed content to cook for me and be there whenever my schedule freed up. I love motorcycles! I love sexy! He embraced almost everything about me. I wanted to believe that could be enough. We didn't share a passion for the same lifestyle, and though I didn't have a clear understanding of my values at the time, I had the nagging sense that ours differed enough to eventually matter. We had fun when we were together, but apart, my mind raced. It wasn't a bad relationship, but it was the wrong relationship. I vacillated between going with the flow and bailing out. I asked everyone I knew – if someone loves and supports you, isn't that all that matters? Why did I need more? He quit smoking – after 23 years. He said it wasn't just for me but still…that had to count for something. I should've loved him for that gesture alone. But of course, I didn't. And I ended it badly without the decency of giving him an honest reason because, at the time, I still didn't completely know it myself.

Though it only lasted for six months, the failure of my relationship with Andy midway through my 40th year threw a cloak of loneliness and depression across my shoulders. I retreated into a two-week cocoon of exile – disconnected, shut down, mourning what I thought to be the death of my most recent relationship, when really it was the unnerving thought that I'd gone down the rabbit hole and again come up empty-handed. Another question mark on the San Francisco horizon, no matter the reasons why. Another person, who I imagined would have an incredible and devoted girlfriend in no time – what might have been mine if I'd been happy enough with what I had.

Being 40 and single presents the increasing awareness that I might be single the rest of my life.

This revelation is, of course, completely unscientific and generally irrational, but when I'm most vulnerable, it strikes me down like lightning, quick and sharp. I contemplate how I veered so far off track to have gone through life so completely undesirable. As my therapist would say, this is a cognitive distortion on my part, but in such moments, I see only the pinnacle of abject relationship failure.

Sometimes I think it might be easier to have fewer passions and interests; fewer expectations and dreams. Easier on a relationship. Easier for starting a relationship. If my interests were simpler – meet man, marry man, buy home, make baby – maybe I'd have it all right now. Why do I feel predisposed to want more? Meet man, go heli-skiing, travel, build mountain home, surf in Mexico, rent apartment in Paris, learn to play guitar, get engaged, go to Bali, maybe marry. I worry that my interests run interference with my love life. Then I worry that maybe I'm just risk-averse. But then I think, if I met someone like me, I'd fall completely in love – what an adventure! And then again, I consider that, quite possibly, I'm the only one who could handle me. And then I get depressed.

It doesn't help that my aging has coincided with a rise in online dating, singles events and the popularity of Dr. Phil, The Bachelor and books on meeting men. I've picked up books like *How Not to be Single* and *He's Just Not That Into You*. They're amusing – good for girl talk – and they offer some sense that I'm being proactive in my attempt at better self-awareness. I'm aware that I'm single and aging. I'm aware that the guy at the bar was definitely not looking at me. I'm aware that while my life feels full, there's an unmistakable void. I've decided that you can make a lot of money writing about meeting men.

The problem for me with much of the advice circulating is the directive to "put yourself out there." Avoid routine, get out of the house, be a joiner. I could fill out my entire Match.com profile just listing activities where one might meet men. I've done dozens of them. Not necessarily to meet men but because they genuinely interested me. In the back of my mind, I thought something might pop up along the way. You know, "Do what you love and the rest will follow?" The rest, the relationship, the happily-ever-after and so on? I've taken meditation lessons and guitar lessons, joined hiking groups and fishing trips, volunteered at sporting events, and weight-trained at gyms across the Bay Area. I belong to a triathlon club, surf (in the noticeably male-dominated waters), and join a ski house every winter. I've signed up for wilderness rescue classes, project management classes and writing classes. I've traveled on my own to Jackson Hole, Greece and Argentina. I've played on softball teams, ultimate Frisbee teams, basketball teams and volleyball teams. I accept invitations to house-warmings, birthday parties, dinner parties, picnics, showers, barbecues, book clubs, art openings, sporting events, and happy hours. I check out as much live music, plays, book readings, wine-tastings, and street fairs as my cultural window allows. I haven't met anyone in the dating pool, but I've put in enough laps to have killer arms.

But is there a point when the activities in my life to "put yourself out there" inhibit my being available for a relationship? When they serve more as a distraction? I'm invigorated by having so many interests and choices that leave me little time to dwell on being single…at least until I'm standing still or contemplating life from my bed, or watching my friends fall in love, all of which I try to avoid.

Coincidentally, at the same time that I've been in overdrive filling the void of my non-dating life, friends who've been lifelong singles are now in serious committed relationships dropping "we" right and left. Their friends are now "ours," certain restaurants are now "special" and Saturdays are sacred date nights. How did this happen? How did every last single person I know find someone? (And do all single people feel this way?) On my darkest of days, I wrap myself in a blanket of bitterness and envy, watching the whirlwinds of new romance swirl all around me, waiting for the moment to pass.

This is my struggle: I want to have a successful, enduring relationship, and I fight the fact that I'm bereft without one. I may very well be single the rest of my life. Would it be easier to know for sure or to continue to find hope? As I get older – as people pair up, move away, build homes and have babies – I feel the need to assert my independence even more – to prove that I'm okay with that. Part of this is the petulant grade school girl in me, still declaring that she doesn't need anyone. Then there's the dread thought that people may feel sorry for me. Still another part feels the quiet rejection of being excluded from a vast, visible segment of society – those in relationships. It's a fine line between proclaiming self-righteous independence and wanting what everyone else seems to have. I vacillate constantly.

On good days, I feel empowered by the choices I've made and am hopeful that the right relationship is still waiting for me. On bad days, I pray for a time when I won't care so much about being alone. Happiness feels tenuous when I consider my contradictory feelings from one day to the next. One chance encounter could change everything.

I ran into Taylor last weekend at a birthday party. He was a quiet, soft-spoken, guitar-playing surfer when we dated. I was there when he caught his first wave and he was there when I bought my first board. I hadn't seen him in over two years. Hadn't heard about him since a mutual friend told me he'd moved in with a girl less than a year after we broke up. For me, another tailspin, another sucker punch, more tears. What did I let slip by? What did she see that I didn't? I'd romanticized his life, his new girlfriend. And there they stood, not five feet away from me. Engaged now. Buying a home. All the next steps in order. She draped her arms around him and he held her hand in his. They smiled and laughed and looked as happy as any engaged couple should be; the smug happiness I often cringed at. Yet somehow, surprisingly, I was okay. Not buy-you-a-wedding-gift, so-happy-for-you okay, but okay okay. Passable okay. I didn't see someone I was craving to be with, didn't see the person I'd spent hours surfing alongside or listening to play guitar, didn't see his depression or inertia that had plagued our relationship. I didn't consider that he might feel superior, knowing that I was still single for completely obvious reasons such as utter incompatibility. I saw a part of my past and I saw a part of his future. Somehow I was momentarily without ego. And for that brief night, I was okay with exactly where and who I was. I had hope. I had acceptance. I had a girlfriend on either side of me. And I had a really cute bartender bringing me drinks.

Samantha Pinney (41) is a project manager with Oracle Corporation in Northern California. Her work keeps her mostly at a desk where she constructs chastising emails to team members and clients who've dropped the ball. Outside of work, she pursues as much as her free time allows – surfing, running, skiing and triathlons, camping, biking, swimming, writing and knitting. She is determined to fill all available time with activity in the twin hopes of meeting someone and sculpting the body she's always wanted. She has a hard time meditating.

If It Were Only Brain Surgery

By Edie Zusman

*S*he came into my hectic neurosurgery clinic elegantly dressed, her suit perfectly accessorized, her voice soft but deliberate. Even at 73, Irene West was confident that the surgery I proposed to treat the painful and debilitating degeneration of her spine would be worth the rare, but potentially catastrophic risks.

She trusted me. She'd said at one point that she did a lot of research to find the right surgeon and chose me, a young female among a sea of better known males, to be her neurosurgeon. Any woman of my generation who would enter this male-dominated field so rife with ego, she reasoned, had to be superb.

I am grateful that she did, because while I was caring for her she taught me that clearing obstacles and forging new ground without bitterness and outrage was not only possible, but empowering. As it turned out, this petite African American woman whose measured determination had influenced her children to stand tall and proud at a time of great social upheaval became a role model for me, just as I hope to be a role model for young women neurosurgeons who will no doubt face hurdles of their own.

When I was a girl growing up in the 1970s, anything seemed possible. The U.S. Supreme Court and Congress had outlawed discrimination based on gender in education, housing, and even human reproduction. I was blithely sure that the women's movement had paved the way. I could be - no, I *would* be - a neurosurgeon.

The brain fascinated me from the time I was eight. In third grade I made a model of the organ, labeled the cerebrum and cerebellum and taped on it an electroencephalogram to illustrate its wondrous activity. Learning how it worked, why it didn't always work properly, and how to make it work better became my passion, and would become my profession.

Despite my early intellectual curiosity, my mother made sure that I knew that my smarts weren't all that special - everybody has gifts - and what matters is what you do with yours to make the world a better place. Straight A's didn't matter if I wasn't going to do something useful with my talents.

What I didn't realize as an ambitious and academically precocious teenager was that becoming a brain surgeon demanded much more than ambition and superior grades in science. I never guessed that my career choice would be an exercise in compromise. Nor did I know just how infuriating it could be trying to rise to the top of a profession designed, dominated and driven by men.

On paper, I was certainly up for the challenge. While in high school, I was accepted into the accelerated, six-year honors medical program at Northwestern University, which allowed me to start medical school at the age of 19. The plan would ensure that I'd finish my education and still have time to complete my equally ambitious personal agenda – to get married and have children - before age 35! By 1987, I had my medical degree and was eager to bring my talent and drive to a fine university medical center where I would train for my specialty.

Today, 20 years after my entrée into the field of neurosurgery, my story is one of great success and satisfaction. I am filled with memories of patients for whom my expertise and training have been invaluable.

I recall, for example, the single father of three who came to me with a pituitary tumor that was causing him to go blind. Today, he can see, has returned to work, and provides for his children. I'll never forget the man with frequent epileptic seizures who had been turned away by other doctors. I got a letter from him recently. He said he hadn't had a seizure since I removed a portion of the temporal lobe where his seizures originated. That was six years ago. And I remember the woman, in her 70s, with a weak heart and a dangerous blood clot between her brain and her skull. The surgery was considered "heroic" and high-risk. Two years later, she is functioning independently and enjoying life with her family.

But my professional success has come at a price. Thinking that 1970s feminism had paved my way, I hadn't bargained for the pervasive barriers that could still prevent women from reaching their potential.

Looking back, I know the bumps I encountered along the road toward neurosurgery were in view even before I'd finished medical school. During one rotation, a department chairman at a West Coast medical school volunteered to write letters of recommendation to neurosurgery programs for me, but refused to accept me into his own program. "You are one of the best students we've had, but I won't be able to accept you," he said. "The other guys just aren't ready to train a woman yet."

Interviews for residency training were equally challenging. The neurosurgery chairman at one top-flight university, for example, asked me how long I could operate without needing to urinate. I'd just assisted on a 14-hour brain tumor surgery without a break, while the male surgeon in charge had taken two.

Not all of the sexist behavior I faced in those days was as subtle. There was the staff member at a prestigious eastern school who, impressed by my research experience, said he would like me to work with him in his laboratory, then slid his hand along my thigh under the table.

Fortunately, I was too determined to be distracted from my pursuits. Besides, I was young and naïve at the time, and I was sure the discriminatory treatment would stop just as soon as I had the credential, as soon as I was among their ranks.

For many years, I thought that to be treated like an equal in neurosurgery I'd have to *look* like a neurosurgeon. So I pulled my long brown hair back, donned clunky glasses and wore a starched shirt with cufflinks under my lab coat. I hoped that by neutralizing my gender, my technical abilities and patient care skills would become the focus, squelching any bias.

In hindsight, it made little difference. Even after 20 years performing craniotomies, removing brain tumors and probing for the source of epileptic seizures, the slights continued. But they only strengthened my resolve to succeed, and to encourage the next generation of women entering my field. That means freely offering my personal phone numbers and email address to medical students and residents who need encouragement or advice at any point along the way. It means housing young researchers on rotation at my home. It means advocating on their behalf when they face discrimination or other obstacles.

There have been breakthroughs. I was the first female neurosurgeon at several universities. I started the brain tumor program and epilepsy research centers at the University of California, Davis. I was president of Women in Neurosurgery, the leading professional organization for women neurosurgeons, and was the first woman neurosurgeon in the 75-year history of the American Association of Neurological Surgeons to serve as a board member.

Today, I hold a full voting post at the AANS, and topping our agenda is the dire need to increase the numbers of applications from women and minorities for neurosurgery residencies to keep our profession thriving. Now that I have walked through the door, my role is to hold it open for others. Some of the same men who'd obliviously undermined my foray into the field now sit at the table with me, looking for ways to attract more women into neurosurgery. Today, for the first time in its history, the association has a sexual harassment clause enabling women to be heard when they experience some of the same things I encountered earlier in my career.

Yet, proud as I am about reaching these milestones and earning my credentials, I don't display the plaques and certificates outside my office door, as some of my male colleagues do. Instead, they adorn my more private, interior office walls, serving as my own necessary reminder of what I've accomplished.

Just as I keep my awards and plaques concealed, so too have I hidden my power, using it quietly in the background to move my very ambitious agenda forward. Ironically (and by necessity), exerting influence over 21st century neurosurgery has demanded behavior reminiscent of a 1950s housewife.

I've learned, for example, that my ideas and bold suggestions for our hospital system will have a greater chance of success if a male colleague presents the plan. I am learning the value of such problem-solving strategies, which ultimately earn recognition and respect through more subtle navigation.

I've learned, too, how to deal with those patients who - unlike Irene West - may have looked at me, politely expressed thanks for explaining the procedure and then insisted on talking with the "surgeon." These days, before we have the first office visit, every patient receives a fancy folder that includes a brief synopsis of my accomplishments. By the time they arrive, they are more likely to appreciate my expertise, and we can get down to business.

I have succeeded in growing my practice as a surgeon, using my talent and expertise to save and extend lives. I am grateful to Mrs. West for her instinctive faith in me, and for sharing her family's story, to help me grasp the idea *that bias is a sign of an evolving society, not a signal to surrender.* She helped a generation to see beyond race by raising strong children and participating in the process. Just as she learned the value of remaining engaged, so have I. I am helping my generation (and inspiring the next) to see beyond gender by staying involved, joining boards, connecting with doubters, and by telling my story. And while I'm proud that I've been able to reach my career goals, I hope that women in the future can fulfill their dreams without having to endure bias. I look forward to the day when my experiences stop being the norm, and instead become an historical footnote.

Edie Zusman (44) is Director of adult neurosurgery at the Sutter Neuroscience Institute in Sacramento. She is recognized as one of the leading female neurosurgeons in the United States. She is active in several leading neurosurgery organizations and was the first woman neurosurgeon on the board at the American Association of Neurological Surgeons. Edie lives in California with her husband, son, daughter, and dog, Lucy. She is quick to point out that motherhood is a lot tougher than brain surgery.

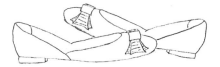

My Most Dysfunctional Relationship

By Esther Gulli

*M*y thirties were exceptionally difficult for me – three miscarriages, the death of my brother John from a drug overdose, a cross country move to a new city with no friends, a major career change and subsequent layoff, two complicated (but thankfully successful) pregnancies, and motherhood. And through it all, food was my constant companion, my drug of choice, seeing me through the emotional meat grinder that had become my life.

As I entered my 40s, I felt as if I was crawling out of a dark cave. All the drama of my 30s was behind me. I had a wonderful husband and two amazing daughters, and I was no longer burdened with the dual mental tortures of trying to get pregnant or maintain a pregnancy. I also had a job I liked, and had managed to find some great friends to stand in for the sister and girlfriends I'd left behind on the East Coast. With all the darkness of my 30s behind me, I was incredibly optimistic about my 40s, and appreciative of the quiet, happy life I was finally living. There was only one cloud hanging over this utopia – the final frontier, my weight.

When I went through grief therapy after my brother's death, which came two days after miscarriage number two, I remember this being the one issue that was absolutely off limits. I told my therapist I wasn't interested in talking about it, and could we just stick to the real issues like death and infertility, blindly oblivious to the interconnectedness of my pain, my grief and my ever-expanding waistline. In retrospect, I expect that it was obvious to him that I was self-medicating with food.

To be sure, I didn't gain all my weight in California. After all, I was born in Tennessee, and spent most of my youthful summers in Mississippi feasting on Aunt Millie's cornbread, black-eyed peas cooked in bacon fat, steak fried up in the black skillet, caramel cake and homemade ice cream – and that was just lunch! My life has been a series of trips up and down that digital scale. But somehow, after moving to the Bay Area – the fit capital of the world – home of organic food, great weather and perfect-bodied people, I managed to gain even more weight and become my largest, most slovenly self.

On or around my 40th birthday in the spring of 2006, I had a conversation with my older sister Elizabeth about how much more difficult it is to lose weight once you hit that mile marker. I also vaguely recall some vow I made about getting down to 140 when I turned 40. It was, of course, an empty promise I had absolutely no intention of keeping.

I think every fat girl has her *aha* moment. That moment when you first see yourself as others must, but somehow you've managed never to let yourself see – through such tricks as well positioned mirrors that either tilt to minimize your hips, or are placed high so as to only show the top (aka good) half of your body.

For me, my stunning moment of recognition came later on that year, when I saw a video of my backside square dancing at family camp with my kids. Now, you'd have to know me to appreciate the utter hilarity of that statement – camping and square dancing are not really two activities that I engage in with any regularity.

But I can still remember the pants I was wearing, how they looked in the video, and how shocking that was for me to see. When I saw that image, all I could think of was how I had so carefully selected those pants that morning because of their "slimming" effect. Clearly, I had stopped living in reality a long time ago. There just aren't a whole lot of places to hide 208 pounds on a frame that's 5'2.

It was horrific. I think there may have even been an audible gasp upon my viewing of this home movie, and to add insult to injury, I knew that my thoughtful friend Eric, who had so lovingly captured this and other sentimental moments from the weekend, had also thoughtfully distributed copies of this creature feature to many of my closest friends.

And there it was, my defining moment. It was quite humbling and effective. The next week, I rejoined Weight Watchers. Like many of the folks around the room, it wasn't the first time I'd been a member. Sadly, I'd been doing this drill since adolescence. I can remember the utter agony of being sent there when I was in junior high. I was the only one under 50 I think, or so I felt. (And that was back in the day when they MADE you eat liver. Could anything be more vile and disgusting?)

Thankfully, just as I have had a series of reinventions throughout my life, so has Weight Watchers. It's come a long way in the last three decades… liver is no longer mandatory, and the leader who told me "bread is your friend" in the '90s has also been corrected. Now they've got that hot, hip, former Duchess to inspire us – *hey, I got dumped by a Prince and the whole world knows it, but look how hot I am now!* I came back to the fat girl club because I knew it was the only way to get me to focus on learning the fundamentals of a healthy relationship with food.

This time, it's been a little different. For starters, I'm still going after a year, when before I think my record may have been four months. I'm there almost every Saturday morning at 7 am. Our leader, Mia, rocks – how else could she get folks there at that God-forsaken hour. And the group itself is an eclectic and inspiring lot. I see recognition in their eyes – even though we're not all in the same place on the journey, we share a lot of the same pains, and we are genuinely happy for each other's successes.

This time, although vanity may have gotten me in the door, I've been more inspired by the prospect of getting healthy so I can be an active mother and do things with my kids like run, hike, and swim. I want to live a long and healthy life so I can see what kind of people my two daughters will grow up to be.

Now, in all honesty, once the weight started coming off, I sure didn't mind that I was looking a lot better. I've started caring more about my appearance. I get my roots done more regularly, to avoid that "continental divide" look. And for the first time in my life, I actually enjoy shopping. Amazing how going from a size 18 to a size 8 can do that for you.

About 30 pounds in to my weight loss journey, I met a blessed angel at Nordstrom, the expert bra fitter, Erica. She gave me my first fitting in probably 25 years, not counting the nursing bra which absolutely does not qualify as anything remotely close to an uplifting experience. God bless Erica…she took me out of a 38C and landed my girls in a 34D, taking fifteen years off my saggy rack. It's amazing how much better your clothes look with breasts that aren't hanging down to your elbows.

And with the top half conquered, I turned my focus to the bottom half and went WAY outside my comfort zone in an attempt to rid myself of the dreaded VPLs (visible panty lines). Acting on a tip from some of my more stylish girlfriends, I finally worked up the nerve to purchase my first thong, a pair of Hanky Pankies. I regret that I was in my fortieth year of life before I learned about these little miracles. The next day, I was back at the store buying eight more. These little lace ditties have transformed my wardrobe. And just last month, I bought my first pair of hip-hugging jeans. I don't even recognize myself anymore.

So yes, there have been some great benefits to losing 48 pounds. I have never felt more healthy and alive. And without a doubt, I *love* that I look and feel better at 41 than I did at 35. Turning 40 was actually a great and wonderful thing. It inspired me to finally take on the challenge of dealing with my most dysfunctional relationship – the relationship with my oldest lover and friend, food. After more than 40 years together, we've finally discovered a way to peacefully co-exist for a long and healthy ever-after.

———————

Esther Gulli (42) works in Student Affairs at a major university. Originally from Tennessee, she set out for Washington DC after college with no job and four cardboard boxes containing all her worldly belongings. She worked in politics for 12 years, including the Clinton White House, and traveled extensively throughout five continents before heading west in 2000. She is married with two kids, and stays in touch with her fabulous network of women. She recommends that all women get a bra-fitting and a pair of Hanky-Pankies as a rite of passage into their 40s.

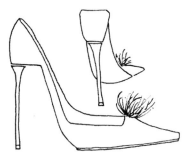

A Cliché Saved My Life

By Vicki Larson

Who's that?" my 17-year-old son asks me. He and his younger brother peer over my shoulder as I flip through the pages of a family photo album.

"Who do you think?"

"I have no idea. Aunt Liz?"

"No silly, it's me."

"Eww! What did you do to your hair?"

It's tough explaining the questionable hair choices of one's youth. Well, I know full well what I did to it; *why* is another matter.

"It's a perm. I used to like those. Why?"

"Ugh. Your hair looks messy," the 17-year-old says.

"Yeah," the 14-year-old chimes in. "It looks like it's fried or something."

They were right. More than just my hair was messy and fried back then. I was in my 30s in the photo, a former career woman adjusting to the world of full-time suburban motherhood for which nothing quite prepared me. I looked like a grown up, despite the juvenile decisions I had made about my hair; I had a beautiful husband, I had two beautiful kids, I lived in a beautiful house, I drove a ... well, a shiny new minivan.

Looking back on that woman more than a decade later, I realize I don't really know who she was. And that's because she didn't know who she was. It took a Big-0 birthday and the transformation into a cliché — a 40-something divorced mother — for me to understand. I was horrified with this new label; as middle-aged clichés go, it is perhaps the biggest of them all. The only way I could have made it worse was if I had studied for a Realtor license, become a family therapist or run off to either Provence to buy a villa or to India to find myself.

A few years earlier I had turned 40. I didn't dread turning 40. I always hated the "9" years more: 29, 39. They signaled the end of something, whereas the "0"s could be seen as the start of something new. Maybe it was just my mind playing tricks on me, convincing me all was going to be okay (like it does when it validates my belief that eating that second slice of chocolate mousse cake is boosting my antioxidant intake rather than padding my hips).

So I thought I'd be able to accept it as easily as I marked my 40th birthday — no party, no fanfare, no ostentation — surrounded by my husband, relieved that he didn't have to plan for a big blow-out party, a 2-year-old still in Pampers and a 5-year-old who wanted to be a Power Ranger. True, it was in Hawaii, but that's where we spent every summer because my husband taught a six-week class at the university there. To celebrate, I slurped down a Mai Tai, threw on a lei, slathered on suntan lotion and packed an extra diaper as we headed to the beach.

Back home, a few soon-to-be-40 girlfriends swept me away for a spa day. As one of the oldest, I was the guinea pig and they watched me carefully — what is 40 like? I may not have been the best of role models, as I still acted pretty much like the giddy teenager I felt like inside. But as we sat in the huge hot tub, feeling fresh and firm from massages and facials, we acknowledged the reality of what we would be dealing with in the years ahead: our Cosmo mags would be replaced by More; PMS by perimenopause; baby sonograms by mammograms; plunging necklines by turtlenecks; natural hair color by a dye (isn't that what they mean when they ask, "Is that your natural color?" Yes, in fact it was my natural color — when I was 9); and our husbands, we feared, would replace some of us with younger, sexier, blonder versions of ourselves.

The only bright spot in getting older, we figured, was the rumored sexual peak that happens to women around 40, and we held onto that hope. True, we were married — we could have sex whenever we wanted! But we weren't really getting much sex and sometimes we didn't even care. We were tired. Sometimes, we were resentful. We didn't even feel all that sexy. Often, we were confused — we were told we could do all and be all, and we sort of believed it. At least, we wanted to. We just didn't fully grasp what that might mean.

Like many women who've gone the distance in a marriage — 14 years — and motherhood, I had given up parts of myself. It happened in such a slow, seemingly innocuous way, that I almost couldn't tell. But I was a willing volunteer; I was a mother, a wife, a homeowner.

All of these required sacrifices. The young woman who'd been out hiking, biking, kayaking, camping, painting, dancing, going to the theater, reading books other than by Dr. Seuss and Dr. Spock, was missing. I'd slowly let go of the things I loved to do because I was too busy doing other things (like making 25 red construction paper roses for a third-grade Valentine's Day party or driving the PTA meeting/ grocery store/dry cleaner/Little League-Boy Scout-soccer-practice route). I didn't regret it — I realized it's just what moms do.

I wasn't necessarily unhappy, or even all that restless; or if I was, I was too busy to notice. Plus, my husband and I appeared to be a happily married couple, and it often felt that way, too. I didn't mind being married and a stay-at-home mommy, even though I had morphed into something unrecognizable from the girl I once was. Even though I never quite felt comfortable saying I was "just" a housewife and mother of two rambunctious boys when asked, "So, what do you do?"

I'd like to say that I had an epiphany, a visit from some sort of spiritual guide, or a visualization that would usher me into my next phase. Or even that I had sought out life coaches or mentors to guide me into the next decade. One in which my growing boys would no longer need me so much, and how that would change my life and my relationship with my husband.

Instead, I was smacked across the face with it by the discovery of my husband's infidelities. Just call me housewife, mother, fool.

There was no way that I could have anticipated how a life I had spent fifteen years building could unravel so quickly. Well, let's just say there's nothing quite like a good old-fashioned crisis to wake you up from the "Groundhog Day" of being a minivan-driving suburban soccer mom.

All my busyness stopped, and I went into survival mode. There were long stretches where all I did was cry, talk to shrinks and read self-help books, months during which I couldn't sleep or eat. Not quite what I thought my 40s would be like as I sat spa-side just a few years before. On the plus side, I'd dropped 15 pounds and everyone told me how great I looked. Looking back, I don't necessarily recommend the Divorce Diet, but it definitely does work. Still, I panicked — who would want a 40-something woman with two young kids?

As fate would have it, a 20-something did. He didn't want me forever — he wanted to eventually get married and have babies with a younger version of me. But he did want me. And against what I would have thought was my better judgment, I wanted him, and not forever either. He was just a little more than a decade older than my oldest son, and I had just gotten out of what I thought would be "forever." My connection with this 20-something was spiritual, intellectual and, yes, sexual, although I'm not sure two romps really count all that much. It was a rebound fling. But what was unspoken was this: someone found me attractive at the exact time that I was feeling most unattractive; someone found me exciting while another saw me as routine; someone thought I had something to say while another saw me as a nag; someone saw me as a sensual woman to explore and delight in while another would rather sleep — or sleep around.

So my new clichéd life as a 40-something divorced mother added yet another clichéd dimension — the younger man. I had to ask myself if I had somehow become a character in a chick-lit book, and a marginally written one at that.

But my fling helped soften the world that had crumbled around me — my marriage exploded right after 9/11, right when my dearest friend moved with her family across the country, right when everyone I wanted to hold close had other ideas. Were my 40s going to be the decade of loss?

Oddly enough, it became the decade of discovery. While the divorce unearthed an inner strength I didn't realize I had, my brief love affair gave me the gift of confidence. I realized I'd been given a chance to get to know who I was in my 40s, irrespective of a partner, now that "housewife" had been stricken from the list — even though, sadly, the minivan remained.

This couldn't have happened at a better time. If I were in my 20s or 30s, I might have been looking for a man to be husband and father, instead of looking for "me." But it happened in my 40s, with just enough of "been there, done that" in me to focus on what I really want. I'm no longer looking for someone with whom to set up house; I have my own house. I'm not looking for someone with whom to make babies; I have my kids. I no longer feel the need to define myself by the love I give — and get — from someone else. Although it's nice to think I may find a life partner, if he never shows up, well, I know I can make it — happily — on my own.

Of all the silly things I bought and did to feel better about being a 40-something divorced mother post-Boy Toy, confidence has been the keeper. I know my body, I know what turns me on, and I know my good side for a photo. I know how to put things in perspective — the house doesn't have to be spotless before I throw a dinner party, my kids won't suffer some horrific disease if they don't eat fruit or vegetables with every meal, and not everyone needs to like me.

That doesn't necessarily mean I haven't made a few bad choices. And it doesn't mean I don't get frustrated with my changing body, miss the smell and comfort of waking up next to a warm body every morning, fret about that age spot that wasn't there yesterday, or question if I should still be shopping in the junior department. But confidence has helped me get real about myself, the world and my place in it, and that's pretty sexy. Maybe that's the sexual peak 40-something women experience.

I don't know what my 40s would have been like without all the drama. Would I have eventually found myself again? Would something else have triggered that confidence? Would I have continued on as a vaguely happy middle-aged minivan-driving soccer mom? I don't know.

But I do know that as I head into the next few Big-0 decades, when things become a little more serious for a woman, I'm counting on that confidence to keep me grounded and help me embrace all that those decades will offer — whether it's retiring in a tiny Italian village, bouncing grandkids on my knee, or trading in the lacy thongs for granny panties.

And who knows — it might even mean that I revisit perms. If I do, however, there will be nothing messy or fried about them.

Vicki Larson (51) is still the mother of two rambunctious boys, who just happen to be taller than she is, and so now she's nicer to them. When she's not fretting over their missed curfews and driving skills, she has worked for almost every newspaper in the Bay Area and has freelanced for numerous publications and Web sites. Now she loves her work at the Marin Independent Journal, where she's the Lifestyles Editor. Surrounded by the beauty of Marin County, she's finally back to hiking, biking, kayaking, dancing and reading, and is living out a childhood fantasy by being the lead singer in a chick band, Sounds Like China. Before that, her biggest claim to fame was having one of her jokes published on the same page as Jerry Seinfeld and Rodney Dangerfield.

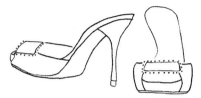

Finding Friendship at Forty

By Cari Shane Parven

I spent my childhood surrounded by estrogen: my mother, my dog, my teachers, and the 42 female classmates with whom I spent first through twelfth grade. There was a little testosterone, floating in the puddles of urine – my brother's pee – that I stepped in (in the bathroom) every morning before school, and in the rings of my father's pipe smoke wafting through our New York City apartment. Other than that, the first half of my life was all about women.

Yet two decades later, as I slid toward 40, excited to celebrate this brand new segment of my life, I found I had no female friends, good friends, to cheer me on. I was happily anticipating turning 40 because it was going to be my decade. Whereas the 20s had been about creating my family – finding my husband, marrying him, and having kids – and the 30s were about staying home to raise those kids, the 40s were going to be about me.

But I was alone. Friendless. I stood in my house considering my life, conjuring up the images of all the women I had known, counting up the years we'd been together, then counting up the years we hadn't been together and then wondering what had happened. Up until that moment I had not seen my lack of good friends as a problem. But as 40 approached – "half way to 80," I would say – I found myself searching for that elusive something that I wasn't getting from my husband and children. Instinctively, I knew what was missing – friendship. I even knew where to find it. The problem was that I didn't have it.

So, why didn't I have friends? I mean I'm no ogre. I love people, I love meeting people, and I actually make friends quite easily. I love the Barbara Streisand song, "People," and I don't find it one bit embarrassing to admit that I even have part of the lyrics, "people who need people are the luckiest people in the world" emblazoned on my high school yearbook senior page. My husband likes to say of me, "she could make a friend in a phone booth."

Yet there's a line between friend and good friend or best friend, and I'd failed at "good" and "best." I never learned how to take friendship up a notch. I lacked follow through, and thus I lost all – if not most – of my friends. Friendship, you see, is an investment of time and self. I hadn't known that. It took me four decades to find that out.

As a child I went to a small school; I had the same group of girlfriends for twelve years. There wasn't much work involved in maintaining friendships then. It didn't take a lot of effort to stay in touch, to see each other and hang out. My best friends and I saw each other everyday at school and, growing up in Manhattan, if I wanted to see them after school or on the weekends, all I had to do was walk a few blocks from my apartment to theirs. It was easy.

When I went away to a small college, I made new friends. Again, it was easy. I had loads of female acquaintances, but now most of my good friends were men. Having grown up in an all-girl environment, I think I was hungry for male companionship. But male friendship doesn't generally work out in the long run. Remember what Harry said, in *When Harry Met Sally*: Men and women can never really be just friends because sex always gets in the way. I actually understand what he meant. Some of my male friends had unrequited crushes on me; others I had unrequited crushes on. One by one, my male friends lost their hearts and attention to their girlfriends. I had invested so much time in my male friendships that by the time I graduated from college I hadn't found that female pal I hoped I'd have forever.

I hardly noticed at the time because I still had the truest friends a girl could ever want: my childhood friends. We were all back in the city, a pre-Sex and the City bunch, meeting for brunch on Sundays, and in bars and restaurants during the week. It lasted for years until we scattered like the wind starting our careers and families. With no Internet to help us keep in touch, we used snail mail and phone conversations. I wasn't one for the telephone, and eventually found that the calls dwindled until they were few and far between. But again, I hardly noticed because I was falling head over heels for my future husband. He filled the void left by my childhood friends and so I didn't realize that I'd let my best friends in the world slip away. I sailed through my 20s energized by the love and affection of my dream guy.

My 30th birthday came and went without much fanfare. I was in the throws of motherhood with a one-year-old and a newborn. Other than an elaborate dinner with my husband, celebration was out of the question. I was busy and not yet aware that besides lacking sleep, I was lacking friendship. After all, I had my husband.

"Who's your best friend?" my children would ask me when they learned to talk.

"Daddy," I'd say proudly, truly proud to call my husband my best friend. I loved the way it sounded. To my ears, it made me seem better than those women who didn't consider their husband their best friend. I believed I needed no more than my husband to fill me up emotionally. I believed that he was my true "BFF" and that he understood me as no female ever had.

"No!" they'd scream. "Daddy is your husband, who's your best friend?"

My children asked me this question over and over through the years, ad nauseam as children do. Then, over time, the answer, the realization, crept into my consciousness: I didn't have one. I didn't have a true best friend. I had abandoned woman-kind.

I had let my friends down. I had, in actuality, been a bad friend. I used my dislike of the phone as an excuse for my limited capacity to follow up and follow through. I was a friend who remembered birthdays but forgot to send a card or make a call. I was a friend who failed to send condolence notes because I wasn't sure what to write, when the words really didn't matter. I was a friend who failed to bring dinner to a friend who really needed a homemade meal.

The realization was hard to take. It actually took years to digest and felt a lot like acid reflux – painful and a recurring reminder of what I'd lost. But as with any kind of pain, you either live with the discomfort or do something to feel better. So, the night before my 40th birthday, I made a resolution. I committed myself to finding friends and figuring out how to build them, keep them, and invest in them.

I went straight to my childhood friends to plead my case and discovered babies who had been born when I hadn't even known of pregnancies; parents who had died when I hadn't even known of illnesses; degrees that had been earned, jobs that had been lost, and moves that had been made. I got on the phone and got an earful. I got on the phone and promised to be there, in sickness and in health, in good times and bad, as long as we both shall live, and I meant it.

In the three years since my resolution I have fostered four fabulous friendships. Doesn't sound like much, but it's actually a lifetime for me – one from every decade of my life. I have many acquaintances, as I always did, but I have four friends (one from my childhood, one from my college years, one from early parenting and one from the present day) upon whom I can rely. And I'm learning how to let my friends rely on me. Because they are so wonderful, because they are such good friends, they are willing to stand by me while I learn even if it means yelling at me because I have forgotten to call them back – again. I still hate the phone but I've learned to multi-task by bringing my cell on walks with the dog. I've also realized that even if I don't feel like talking at the exact moment a friend has called, she might be the one who needs me. I've learned to text, which is a fast, easy way to stay in touch and of course, I'm madly in love with e-mail – a brilliant form of communication.

What I have found is that these friends, these four amazing women, fill an indescribable void that can't be filled by my family.

It's a void children can't fill because they are natural takers. It's a void a husband can't fill because no matter how in touch he is with his "feminine side," the fact is that men just don't think, listen or talk like women. So, as I slide through the fourth decade of my life I see how I've come full circle, back to the comfort of my early estrogen nest. It's a wonderful, comfortable place held together with love and companionship, understanding and commiseration. It lacks judgment and is overflowing with support. It's a security net woven of women, by women and for women.

Cari Shane Parven (42) is a former television reporter, based in Potomac, Maryland. Her perfect day would include a morning swim, a day of skiing (preferably in Montana) and an evening on her laptop writing about human behavior. Her dream as a child was to be like Jane Goodall sitting in the forest among the chimps or Margaret Mead observing the natives in Samoa. As a mother of three and wife to one, she can do neither. So instead, she blends into the culture around her and writes about what she sees. Her observations can be found in her two blogs, Inside the Beltway and Under the Radar and Keepin' It Real.

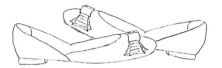

What A Long, Strange Trip It's Been

By Lauren Bogart

On the evening of my 40th birthday I had a teary one-way conversation with my deceased husband. Tinged with guilt and regret, I bid him yet another painful farewell as I entered a decade that he never had the privilege to reach. He will be eternally young, having passed away at age 38. He lived half a life. I reminded him that we were supposed to spend the next half together.

Our family had finally reached a point where there are no more middle of the night feedings, diaper changes and ear infections. It seems unfair. Why aren't you here with us, Paul? What fun the five of us would be having at this precious stage. We should have been marking the milestone of my 40th together – planning our future and all the wonderful things which lay ahead – Bar Mitzvahs, graduations, weddings, grandchildren, retirement and travel. We were supposed to grow old together. As I considered these missed milestones, I was keenly aware that turning 40 is a privilege, not an entitlement, and I felt a bit robbed.

The family unit, myself included, is growing up, but we are missing a key component who, in most ways, is irreplaceable. Who else would have the same twinkle in his eye when our children make us proud? Who else would share my concern over the silly things that parents obsess over?

Our lives changed on February 13, 2002. I was five months pregnant with our third child, and Paul was diagnosed with a brain tumor. What had been a nagging headache for the prior couple of months suddenly became a death sentence. While doctors tried to be positive and offered various treatment options which ultimately failed, it was understood that without a cure, Paul would not survive the tumor. I walked the halls of the hospital that day thinking it was my own personal 9/11. The following two years were hideous in countless ways. We rode an emotional roller coaster. Stress levels and optimism rose and fell based on MRI results. We were exhausted – he from his treatments and me from running a household which included two children, a newborn baby and a sick husband. Yet during the 21 months that Paul's tumor was kept at bay, we held out some hope that a cure was around the corner. As unlikely as it was, I allowed myself to dream that our lives could, one day, return to normal.

Just as Paul was finishing his last round of chemo, we were broadsided again. His tumor had returned, in a more critical location of the brain than before, and he needed a second brain surgery. He came out of that surgery grossly impaired, and was never himself again. He became like a fourth child to me. My Wharton-educated husband no longer knew the names of his children. He called me "mom." He couldn't tie his shoes, walk or toilet himself. We lived this way for six months. At age 37, I was a widow.

This was not a shock, of course. I had been mentally preparing myself for this day since his diagnosis. And yet, there is a finality to death that must be experienced to truly be understood. Despite all the nights at hospice watching for his last breath, when the nurse with the stopwatch proclaimed that the last one had been taken, I felt a blow to my stomach. I remember saying over and over, "He's gone, he's gone," as if trying to convince myself that he really was.

When I walked out of the hospice for the last time, I witnessed the most glorious sunrise I had ever seen. Although I don't consider myself a spiritual person, it reassured me – that Paul was going to a better place and that we, his loved ones, would emerge from this dark period of our lives.

Despite my sadness, I must admit that, over time, I experienced a new sense of freedom. I could feel my age again and not be tied to aides' schedules, doctor's appointments and the demands of Paul's sick mind and body. In short, I was ready to start getting on with my life and raise my kids in a more normal environment.

Life is a big, juicy novel filled with many, many chapters. In my more free-spirited youth, I thought I would write those chapters, fully in control of my destiny and direction. Experience has led me to recognize, though, that fate, luck and other outside forces are contributing authors.

Reflecting back on my life a half lifetime ago, I chuckle. At 20, I was a liberal feminist at the University of Michigan, working hard to get into a top law school. I thought a law degree would enable me to help women escape the economic injustice divorce often brought.

I had seen the consequences of divorce in my own childhood home, watching my mother, who had been a homemaker, struggle to raise her three daughters in the way we had grown accustomed to in a two-parent household. I vowed never to repeat her mistakes – never to give up a career to have children, and never to be economically dependent on a man.

Fast forward: I fell in love with a business school student while in law school, married and had three beautiful children. I veered off course by giving up the big law career and becoming a stay-at-home, minivan-driving mom in the suburbs. I was happy, although tired and stressed like any mom of babies and toddlers. Our marriage was strong, even though it was hard to keep the flames of romance kindled as they had been before we'd had kids.

In the words of Paul's favorite band, "What a long, strange trip it's been." Yet I'm happy. Should I feel guilty saying it? It's not what people expect to hear from a 41-year-old widow and mother of three. I worry that others might think that I didn't love my husband enough. Not true. If I were the sole author of my life story, he'd still be here with us, enjoying his children as they grow into people worthy of his pride.

I'm not into pity parties though. I've recognized from the first day of diagnosis that things could be a lot worse. While Paul was alive, I was able to give him the highest quality of life that his body and mind would allow. Since his death, I have maintained our lifestyle for myself and the kids so that their daily lives continued uninterrupted. We are in the same house. We are surrounded by the same supportive friends and family who buoyed us when we were at our lowest. I am lucky to live in the town I grew up in. I can't imagine having to deal with a spouse's death and single parenting any other way.

My kids kept me going. Even in the hardest times, I never pulled the covers over my head and refused to get out of bed. I couldn't. I had three vulnerable children depending on me. I remember when a hospice worker came for a visit during Paul's illness, I asked her how my children would fare when their father passed away. I'll never forget her answer. "Children do as well as the surviving parent." When I met with the rabbi of my temple to discuss Paul's funeral, he reminded me, "Only one person's life ended today. Not yours." Those words stuck with me.

I am grateful for the strength and resilience I never knew I had. I resolved to be happy, and I am. That effort and attitude is in my control and I protect it fiercely. This attitude has enabled me to find love again. How lucky to have such love – not once, but twice in a lifetime! I am blessed. It seems crazy that a neighbor, who divorced and sold his house five years ago, is now my significant other. If people had described that scenario several years ago, I would have thought them out of their mind. It's just further evidence that we really don't know what the future holds.

The night after marking my upcoming 40th with reflections of Paul and what will never be, I exuberantly celebrated at a party thrown for me by Adam, my wonderful boyfriend of two years, who touched my heart with a beautiful toast and slideshow, and added sparkle to my neck with a diamond necklace. We drank martinis with old friends and new ones, and laughed as we flipped through a scrapbook filled with pictures from my childhood. That evening, we whispered sweet nothings and enjoyed the comfort of knowing that we have the rest of our lives to look forward to.

I am living an amazing new chapter and enjoying it immensely as it unfolds. Our life together is wonderfully chaotic, thanks to the seven kids between us. Somehow, though, with love, respect and patience, we make it work.

When I think about the future, there are many question marks. What I do know, however, is that experiencing a tremendous loss has given me a better perspective than I had years ago. My feathers aren't as easily ruffled and things that once may have worried me now seem trivial. I am more conscious about living in the moment and making memories with my kids, boyfriend, family and friends. It is my challenge and responsibility to keep my husband's memory alive while balancing our need to move forward. I know Paul would approve because, in his unselfish way, he'd want us to be happy. Thankfully, we are.

Lauren Bogart (41) is an attorney who is taking a long "career hiatus" from full-time law while juggling the busy lives and activities of her three children. Previously, Lauren was a healthcare and insurance attorney at a Washington DC-based law firm. Since her late husband was diagnosed with a brain tumor in 2002, Lauren has been actively involved in fundraising for brain tumor research. She is Teams Chairperson of the Race for Hope 5K which raised over $1.7 million in 2008 to support the Brain Tumor Society and Accelerate Brain Cancer Cure organizations. In her free time, Lauren enjoys running, working out, reading, and traveling.

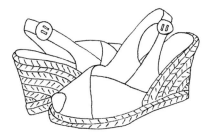

The Imaginary Nursery

By Stephanie Vanderslice

$\mathcal{I}$ have a confession to make. I've been decorating the nursery again.

Some of you will know exactly what I'm talking about, but for those of you who don't, I'll elaborate: the nursery in my mind.

It is a phenomenon that occurs on a semi-regular basis in my life. Something wonky happens with my monthly cycle, something that probably has a lot more to do with the fact that I'm forty-one than anything else, and my mind runs to pastel prints and crib mobiles, to thoughts of "What if. . ."

"But I thought you were done," my friends might say. "I thought you had all you wanted. I thought you weren't even trying."

"Yes," I would answer. "All those things are true – and then some." Like the fact that not only am I forty-one, but my husband is forty-seven and my youngest child is seven. And the fact that this child, who regularly professes a deep longing for a younger brother or sister (in spite of his reputation for refusing to share even a lap) would probably be sent into a tailspin if he were granted his wish and lost his coveted status as the baby of the family. Truth be told, the motivation behind his desire for a younger sibling is somewhat suspect:

"Why do you want a little brother or sister so much?" I once asked innocently.

"So I can tell him what to do," he answered, without missing a beat.

Then there's the fact that, with two boys, we still have a girl's name we're dying to use. And, just in case, a boy's name too.

Finally, there's also the fact, and this one looms fairly large in my nursery daydreams, that I have always harbored a secret desire to be surprised by pregnancy.

Now, if you *have* been surprised by pregnancy, *or* if you're still trying for your first, you might want to stop reading at this point. You're not going to feel very sympathetic to the rest of my confession, and I wouldn't blame you one bit.

I have always envied the highly fertile among us. Both my children, conceived when I was twenty-nine and thirty-three, required a certain amount of worry, hand-wringing, specialist visits and, in the end, a healthy dose of pharmacology, for which I will spend the rest of my life thanking the higher power. Seven years later, we know that a return to "trying" would probably mean even more heartache, and a level of reproductive technology of which we have yet to hear. That, in fact, was why we decided to stop at two. We felt lucky. We felt blessed. Deliberately choosing not to travel once more down that uncertain road, we wanted to end our reproductive efforts on a high note.

154

I used to chastise myself for unrolling those nursery blueprints in my head. "Why," I'd say, mentally rapping my forehead, "do you *do* this to yourself when you know that the chances of your being pregnant at forty-one, having been fertility-challenged your whole adult life, are about the same as your being struck by lighting – twice – *and* winning the lottery?"

The truth is, even with those kinds of odds, I still see plenty of women making these long-shot bets. And some actually pay off. The woman pushing the two-year-old on the playground swing who tells you, grinning sheepishly, that her other "baby" just started college. The older couple you'll never forget encountering years ago in Wal-Mart at Christmas, fawning giddily over a six-month old in a shopping cart. You were sure they were the child's grandparents until they came up out of their love-induced trance long enough to tell you, "We were told we'd never have a baby."

So I've stopped scolding myself. After all, who *doesn't* fantasize about winning the lottery?

We'd probably have to convert the back room. I've done the baby-blue, so I'm thinking a nice, sophisticated taupe print, with dark brown accents. Maybe a little velvet trim. After all, there'll be grandchildren someday, I hope. And they'll need a place to sleep.

Stephanie Vanderslice (41) teaches creative writing at the University of Central Arkansas and often writes about parenting, growing older, and her passion for books in articles, essays and on her blog. She is at work on a novel, *The Secret Baby*. She is proud to be part of a small but growing group of creative writers in higher education trying to shake things up a little, as co-editor of *Can It Really Be Taught: Resisting Lore in Creative Writing Pedagogy* (Heinemann 2006) and author of a number of articles and books on teaching creative writing. A garage and estate sale connoisseur, she lives outside Little Rock, Arkansas with her husband and two sons and happily forks over thirty-five dollars a year to the DMV for a license plate that says "READ2EM."

A Fresh Coat

By Sonia Alison

I turned 40 this year. Actually, I have always enjoyed aging. Ever since I can remember, I have wanted to be older, a "real adult." Being a child was not very appealing to me, but adulthood always looked good. Now here I am. Much to my surprise, I still don't mind getting one year older every year. I don't need things to go any faster but I feel like I squeeze just as much life out of each year as I can, and thus have no regrets. My body is holding up and I'm entering an exciting new phase in my work.

So I was rolling happily along, playing with my style and appearance, delighted to be returning to full-time work now that my child is starting kindergarten, feeling somewhat accomplished and capable. Forty, great! Sexual peak and all that.

Then my husband informed me he wants to end our marriage. So much for rolling along. It was as if I was driving along fairly smoothly in my sedan of life, enjoying the ride, when *BLAM*, I skidded over some ice and careened into a tree, totaling my car. Like an accident victim, I'm now in need of a special mix of physical and emotional therapy, learning how to do things again, but differently (maybe even more intelligently). Wandering down the aisles in the supermarket, I catch myself reaching for items I no longer need to buy. Instead of clashing with an unneighborly neighbor as I might have done before, now I offer a smile and a cup of tea. Now I express gratitude to the people I love more often and more intentionally. I seem to have lost my sense of righteousness, my sense that I know things already. I now approach experiences open to more points of view, open to advice from those who've come before me, open to the quiet wisdom of aligning myself with integrity and compassion from the beginning.

Abruptly, I stopped coloring my hair, cut it short, and stopped wearing make-up. You might think I'm just sad or depressed, but I always wanted to be more natural. I think a lot about our culture's narrow definition of beauty, the influences under which we make decisions about our appearance, and now, of course, what it means to be "an older woman." For many, it's less visible, less desired, less powerful.

Being rejected by my husband at this transitional age was a blow, to say the least. I was supposed to age with him, safe in the knowledge that he loved me, found me desirable, remembered me in my youthful beauty as the rest of the world takes less and less notice. Now what? I have boobs – that might help.

But really, what can I expect? I had a dream last night that I was sitting with my sister (happily married and younger than I am) and a cute, youngish guy, maybe 28. We were outside near a pool or the ocean, some body of water, and I had my bathing suit on, which translates, in my dream interpretation, into ultimate vulnerability. The guy and I are talking and I'm getting the impression that he's, maybe, interested in me, you know, and thinks I'm pretty, sexy – you get the picture. Somehow, in the dream, I find myself asking him, in the course of our flirting, "How old do you think I am?" He says, "60."

I was crushed, mortified, deeply distressed. Here I thought this man was proof that I was still an interesting and appealing woman, someone who could expect to be desired again someday. I don't mean to offend women close to 60 – intellectually I know that women of all ages can be desired – but I guess I felt like a fool, *such* a fool. Maybe that's the message of the dream: at 40, as an object of desire, I feel like a fool.

What's great about 40? I don't give a shit, anymore. Almost. So what if salt and pepper hair isn't the most flattering color for me? I want my entire house painted yellow inside. I can let my daughter eat before she's washed her hands. These aren't my most radical sentiments, of course, but I'm beginning to feel less constrained by "shoulds." I'm noticing this new state of being: uncontained, uncorked, unleashed. I am now detached from specific outcomes, and instead, float just above the certainties in which I used to believe. I do worry, a little, about where this "genie out of the bottle" might lead me, and especially if I am going to embarrass myself, or more likely, embarrass my daughter.

Reading a recent *New York Times Sunday Book Review*, I noticed a trendy new genre – the teenager lusting, almost uncontrollably, for a woman in her 40s. This plot line seems ridiculous and insulting to me. Is it wishful thinking on the part of these 40-something authors?

Are they just trying to sell books to women? How often does this happen in real life? Is this what I want, to have sex with a boy? Is this where feminism has gotten me? I don't think so.

I remember making the decision to have only one child. This was my plan, and for my daughter's first three years of life I was very happy. Then, all of a sudden, I started to stare at pregnant women. I was 38. The force of my unexamined impulse to have a second baby was impressive to me. After months of trying to make sense of this, I realized that I was not wrestling with whether or not I wanted another child, but instead I was struggling to accept aging.

For forty years I have been the youthful princess, fertile in all endeavors. Turning away from fertility felt like walking off a precipice, falling into something unknown, without light. As someone who considers herself a strong feminist, I sheepishly had to admit that I was afraid, sad, and angry that other females would take my place in society's hierarchy. The intense and continual cultural messages about youth were going to be harder to counteract than I'd imagined. At times, I find myself feeling invisible. Everywhere, it seems, moving towards not being counted. Is it important that I am visible? Visible to whom? And for what? This seems to be the work for my 40s. I am making it up as I go along.

Here's my new favorite nursery rhyme for the next decade:
A wise old owl sat in an oak,
The more she heard, the less she spoke;
The less she spoke, the more she heard.
Why aren't we all like that wise old bird?

As a younger woman, I thought I knew a lot about everybody else. As a woman of 40, I feel I know a lot about me, and not much about everybody else. I want to listen more, judge less, and enlarge my own definition of fertility. I want to trust myself and my hard-earned instincts. I also want to paint every room in my house a cheerful yellow...

———————————

Sonia Alison (41) has been an educator for eighteen years. She teaches children in elementary school as well as supports new teachers entering the profession. She has presented at several conferences and received a J. Russell Kent award for her work with young children and gardens. She lives in Northern California and enjoys reading, hiking, and yoga. On her "to do" list is to learn to play the guitar. Although she hasn't painted her house yet, her office welcomes all with a fresh coat of Sundance Yellow.

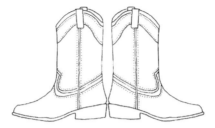

The Weight of Words

By Susan Reinhardt

*I*t was the words. Not the images in the magazines of the gorgeous models weighing all of 108 pounds and wobbling on legs the width of swizzle sticks. The playground chant ends, "but words will never hurt you." But they did.

First from my band director. I was 15 years old, 5'8" and couldn't have tipped the scales at more than 110. One day, as I placed my clarinet next to my Bonne Bell glossed lips, he approached. "You're butt's getting mighty wide," he said, in his South Georgia accent. He winked. His words shattered my fragile teenage self-confidence.

I began jogging every day and skipping lunch at school. I was a cheerleader in a small town in Georgia, fairly popular and attractive in that Farrah-Fawcett-haired way. While my rear-end has always packed a bit of "junk in the trunk," my figure was considered near-perfect by many. I kept my weight down and obsessed over every calorie. During my freshman year of college, I came home after three months away. Home for Thanksgiving, for that wonderful time when families gather and give each other the love and warmth they've saved up just for this special occasion.

The first words from my father's mouth weren't meant to be cruel. But they would leave a devastating impact. "Good Lord, what an arse!" he said. "How much do you weigh?"

He'd told my younger sister and me that men liked thin women. That no decent man would marry a fat woman. My own mother was beautiful and thin, and still is, but not from an eating disorder. She inherited great genetics. I inherited my grandmother's thighs and fanny, as well as her appetite for fried foods and the propensity to pack on pounds.

I went back to college where the real impact of an eating disorder reared its malevolent head. My roommate taught me how to gorge and throw up. She was beautiful, exotic and from a rich family in Buckhead, the swanky section of Atlanta. "You can eat all you want, and if you top it with ice cream, it'll come up much easier."

I began to binge and purge. Not regularly, but occasionally. I also ate nothing but Dexatrim and salads. By the time I returned home at Christmas, my weight had fallen to under 107. People complimented my figure - the destruction grew like a virus with such words of praise.

I transferred colleges and switched from a nursing major to journalism. I also joined a sorority, one of the biggest institutions of eating-disordered behavior I've ever known. Cheerleaders and beauty queens, regular girls with their own inner demons, all gathered in that huge mansion known as our sorority house. But below the hardwood floors and floral-print chairs, the plumbing system carried away the vomit of these Southern belles. I began writing down every single thing I ate and the caloric content. I jogged, did the Jane Fonda-type aerobics so hot in the '80s. I was thin. And I was miserable.

One day during my senior year, I'd had enough. I began eating regularly. The weight returned like iron shavings to a high-powered magnet. "You used to have the best body on campus," a frat boy told me one day. "Why did you go and gain all that weight?"

Words. Words. Words. They were far more damaging than even comparing myself to the beauties on TV who don't weigh enough to give blood.

For years I struggled with food obsession and a love/hate relationship with my body. I had great legs, even as I grew older but the cellulite (also hereditary) began appearing. My ankles were thin, as were my wrists. I hated my upper arms and thighs, but things were better at this point in my 20s. I'd married a man who liked women "with some meat on their bones."

I got healthy and pregnant and gained 40 pounds with each child. After giving birth, I joined Weight Watchers and began to accept that a woman of my height looks perfectly normal and beautiful weighing 135 to 140.

One day an epiphany arrived in the most unlikely source. An old man with cataracts clouding his swimming-pool blue eyes said to me: "Susan, don't nobody want a bone but a dog." Words. Words. His changed my life. He was a simple man with a country accent and a swoop of tobacco dribble in the crook of his wrinkled chin. Something about those eyes mesmerized me. Why was I worrying about my weight when I was just like this man, a regular human being, not some supermodel who had to starve to squeeze into a pair of Victoria's Secret undies?

"Don't nobody want a bone but a dog." He said it. The words. They made perfect sense, and I never forgot them.

I am now a 46-year-old mother of two who wears an array of sizes, depending on the make of clothing. I don't own scales - I threw them out years ago. If I'm hungry I eat. If I see cellulite turning my fanny into a waffle iron, I smile.

Beauty is knowing our bodies have been good to us, despite what we've done to them. I choose to love my shape and have accepted that as I age, it shifts, just like a sack of flour.

No longer do I have "junk in my trunk." Now I'm buttless and the extra pounds are inner-tubing my mid-section. My friends and I can laugh and call it the "meno-pot." It's okay. My arms waddle like pelican pouches with fresh fish flopping inside. That's okay, too.

As I get older, I have come to appreciate the delicious parts of my body, the parts that still work. It's no longer a matter of perfection, but of function. And I'm functioning just fine. Thanks to that old man's words.

Susan Reinhardt (46) is a syndicated columnist, mother of two and author of three books, the most recent being *Dishing with the Kitchen Virgin*. Her first book, *Not Tonight Honey, Wait Til I'm a Size 6*, was a bestseller, and her second book, *Don't Sleep with a Bubba* won a literary award as one of the best books for 2007. She is also a popular public speaker and humorist. Susan now eats a little chocolate every day.

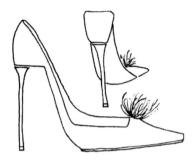

Crisis Tattoo

By Colleen Gregory

When I quit, I had been at the agency for longer than I'd been married. I had thought that I would stay forever; that I would lead the agency when the founders retired. I had been so happy there for so long, that for months and months I denied my creeping unhappiness. Then there was the meeting in which a new executive berated me in front of my solemn, embarrassed peers, while my cell phone rang and rang, ever more insistently. My son had vomited at summer camp and the counselors wanted me to pick him up. I finally extracted myself from the meeting, listened to the camp counselors' increasingly urgent messages, and went to get him. I swore out loud the whole way to camp that I would leave my job as soon as I could. I was surprised by my sudden vehemence.

I started to think about getting my first tattoo. I saw lots of dancers with beautiful tattoos in my weeknight and Saturday morning yoga classes. Years before, after a bad break-up, I had pierced my navel. Somehow, it had helped me to leave some of my sadness behind. Maybe a tattoo would help me to physically mark the end of my first career.

My husband Jay and I decided that I could quit at the end of September, and stay home for a few months while I looked for something part-time. I would help the kids ease into the new school year. I would exercise; I would dance; I would read at the café around the corner. Maybe I would take singing lessons. I would do all the things around the house that had needed doing for the decade we had lived there. I would make some small repairs to the house; I would get us ready for the big Northern California earthquake that everyone said was coming soon.

But instead, I met a man at the café, and I shook the entire foundation of my life.

* * *

Jay and I had been married for 10 years. Recently, I'd been reminding myself how we used to be one of those couples that I now hated to be around – the kind of people who held hands and touched all the time. Where did all that go, I wondered? We didn't fight, but it was very quiet between us. We talked about the kids, the house or our jobs. Sometimes I felt alone, even in the midst of my beautiful little family.

Ford was almost 10 years younger than I; he managed the surf/skateboard shop down the street from my house. He biked or skateboarded to work; he was always a little bit brown, even in December. He saw me with Jay sometimes; he saw me with the children a lot. He said "Hi" to me every day when I went by myself to get coffee before sprinting to the office to be berated by the new leadership. When I quit, and stopped rushing to work every day, he talked to me more. He said, "You seem happier. Are you happier?" One day during the rainy season I walked past the shop in the pelting rain with my hood up, peering in front of me just as he emerged from the shop. "You look cute today," he said. I began to look forward to seeing him; I started noticing his work schedule.

I knew, without admitting anything to myself, that I needed to find other ways to occupy my mind, so I started to look in earnest for a part-time job. I told Ford that it seemed I wouldn't get the job I thought I wanted, and I wasn't able to muster much enthusiasm for the two offers I did get. He said, "It's okay; it just wasn't meant to be. I mean, if you had gotten the job, maybe your boss would have made a pass at you." He smiled and looked at me, oddly expectant. Maybe I imagined that. I asked him, "Has that ever happened to you? Has your boss ever made a move on you?" He laughed and his teeth flashed white against his golden surfer skin. "No, not exactly... But then, I've always been the boss." He paused, then said, "Make a list of all the things that are most important to you in a job; then compare these two jobs against your list."

That sounded simple enough. I dutifully wrote down a list of desirable job characteristics; in my head I made a list of all the things that I liked about Ford. A couple of days later I saw him, and he asked about my list. I told him I'd made two lists and I would tell him about the second one, but he had to promise not to laugh. He stared at me and said, "I could never laugh at you." I pushed out the words, "I made a list of all the things I like about you." I couldn't look at him.

I blurted out, "I have to go to my dance class." I ran away with my heart pounding in my chest.

The next day, Ford said, "We should compare lists." And so we did – we met for coffee on his day off and he asked me what was going on in my life. I told him I was lonely and I didn't know why. I said I loved my husband, but there were no surprises and not much passion anymore. I loved my children but I felt like I was just a mommy and a wife. I missed men looking at me like they used to. I missed feeling beautiful; sometimes when I looked in the mirror I thought I could feel my life draining away. I said more. My parents had died young. My older sister Jana was letting herself go grey. Sometimes, as much as I loved my sister, I was terrified to be around her, to see her aging in front of me. His cell phone rang and he ignored it. He said, "You're being so honest with me. I need to tell you that I have a girlfriend. It's an open relationship and she lives a few hours away." I thought that meant it was ending; I wanted it to mean that it was ending.

We went for a walk and sat down on a secluded park bench, with winter-bare rosebushes all around. He turned toward me and kissed me. I felt electrical impulses shoot through my arms, my legs, my whole body. His tongue slid in to my mouth, and he groaned. Maybe I groaned, too. I kissed him back like I was drowning; when I came up for air, I ran my fingers along his jaw line, his ear, his neck. He said, "I didn't know you were so tactile. You're adorable." He ran his hands around my face, through my hair. "I've been staring at you for months." I asked him, "Did you think about this? Did you think about kissing me?" He nodded. I surprised myself by saying, "I've thought about much more inappropriate things." He laughed, "That could be arranged." His phone rang again. He looked at the number and stood up. He said, "I have to go; we're going snowboarding today." I stood up slowly. I said, "Sitting down was so nice; what would standing up be like?" I stepped into his arms and he kissed me again; he was shorter than Jay. He didn't have to bend down; his left hand reached around my waist and pulled me hard into him. He said, "I really have to go."

I was consumed by waves of intense emotion; I was wracked by guilt. I mustered all of the courage I could find and told Jay that I had a crush on someone. He was stunned. He said, "I don't know what to say. When did this happen?" He didn't look at me for several days. I asked if he would go to couples counseling with me. He agreed, reluctantly. I left the house one evening to walk the dog, and to get away from Jay's hurt, angry face. Ford was leaving work on his bicycle. He stopped to talk to me on a dark side street. I told him what I had done. He inhaled sharply and looked exasperated for a moment. He asked, "Why did you do that?" I said I owed it to Jay to tell him some of what was happening. I continued, "And the only reason that I'm telling you is so that you will know me and understand what is going on with me." He exhaled and stepped closer. "That's all I ever wanted. You know, before I knew your name, I made up names for you. Some days I called you Penelope; some days I called you Katherine." I stared at him. He looked right in my eyes and said, "I love you." I took a sudden breath. I said, "You do?" He said, "I wish I could take care of you." I looked around – there was no one else on the cold, dark street. I kissed him. He said, "We'll talk some more soon," and he got on his bicycle and left quickly and silently.

I was wildly conflicted; I felt horribly guilty. Jay and I started couples counseling but my heart wasn't in it. I tried to go through the motions anyway. Jay wanted me to say at our first session that I was committed to the marriage and that I would do anything to fix what was wrong. I couldn't say it. The therapist said that it was okay not to say it, that it was better not to lie. I felt even worse.

One day, Ford's best friend from the surf shop stopped to pat my dog outside the café. There was a thin sun breaking through the early spring clouds and I was having my coffee outside. He sat down for a moment. Still petting the dog, he glanced at me sideways. He said, "You know Ford's engaged to a woman up in Tahoe? They're getting married in September." I started to pick up my coffee cup, but stopped mid-motion. My arms were tingling and warm. I felt like when I was last pregnant and sick every morning and evening for months on end. I wondered in a distracted way if I was going to faint. My dog sidled over and put his head on my knee; he looked up at me quizzically from under his furry eyebrows. "You didn't know, did you?" I heard Ford's friend ask from some distance away. "No, I didn't know," I was finally able to say. He stood up abruptly and started to go into the café. He turned back for a moment. "I'm sorry, I thought I should tell you," he said.

Later, Ford said, "I told you it was an open relationship. What else could I have said to make you understand?" I stared at him incredulously and said, "But how is it open if you're getting married?" He spoke as if I were a child who needed some simple directions repeated: "I'll have things on the side and so will she. It will still be open." I realized I was staring at him with my mouth agape. I finally said. "But I can't fool around with you if you're engaged." Later I wondered how I could be so self-righteously angry with him for his engagement when all along, I was married with children.

I continued couples counseling and tried harder. The therapist suggested that we do new things together, not just our usual date-night dinner and a movie. I remembered the tattoo. It seemed like years, not months ago that I had considered a tattoo to help me get over my career woes. I suggested that Jay and I get a babysitter and go find a tattoo artist. We went to several shops. We looked through artists' portfolios full of hearts and skulls, buxom women and R.I.P. tributes. We both liked one man's portfolio of birds and flowers and Dr. Seuss tattoos; he agreed to sketch a lower back tattoo for me. If I liked it, he would tattoo the outline in a couple of hours, and then fill in the color a few weeks later.

Our therapist asked us, "How are things at home while you're coming to see me? Do you talk to each other?" Jay said that we weren't connecting; he wondered if he should start planning for the end of the marriage. One day, I overheard him talking to a friend on the phone, "Oh, she's okay, it's me who doesn't know what to do…" Am I okay, I wonder? I am in a strange place in my mind, where absolutes don't seem to exist. I am a little crazy, I think. The only time I can remember living in such a prolonged state of magical thinking was when my mother was sick, only a year after my father passed. I knew my mother was going to die, but sometimes I acted like an ungrateful teenager around her. I knew I would lose her, and I took her for granted at the same time.

A few weeks later, Jay and the kids gave me singing lessons for my birthday. I cried at the dinner table and couldn't stop. My son said, "Mommy, why are you sad?" My daughter said, "Mommy, if you're scared I could go with you. You know that I can sing much better than you can." Jay smiled cautiously and said, "We thought you'd like to try something new." I left the table and went to the bathroom. I blew my nose and tried to stop crying, but soon I was sobbing. Jay followed me and asked if I was okay. I nodded through my tears; I didn't deserve how kind he was to me, even at that moment.

For a long time, I had wanted to really be able to sing. Jay is very musical, and sometimes he visibly winced when I sang. I always knew the words, but I couldn't carry a tune. I knew it was painful for him to hear me, so I stopped singing in front of him. I sang along with CDs in my car – the Beatles, Bob Dylan, James Taylor, Johnny Cash, Patsy Cline.

I started the voice lessons; every week I practiced scales, triplets, enunciation, volume control, breath control. I sang flat, I sang on pitch, I couldn't find the melody, my range stretched out some, I got a little better every week. My teacher taught me how to sing from my chest, to feel the vibration in my body, all the way to my heart, when I did it right.

I decided to surprise Jay's family by doing a short song at his sister's wedding reception in the early summer. The teacher and I picked an old Johnny and June Cash duet; I would do both parts. She warned me, in a kind way, that I might not be ready. Jay was even more careful with me. He said, "You're braver than me, but it would be too bad if you sang and it didn't go well – then you might not want to sing ever again." I told the kids what I was planning; my daughter offered to help me practice. She said, "Mommy, you're getting better, but I still sing way better than you do."

* * *

When Ford and I started to speak again, I told him about the tattoo. He asked, "Where and what?" Another day he said, "I want to see it after you get it done." I looked at him; I couldn't look away. He stared back at me. He said, "Katherine, Penelope, whatever your name is, I want to see it." I felt myself leaning toward him; the dog suddenly pulled me the other direction. I shocked myself by saying over my shoulder, "I want to show you."

I got the tattoo outline. Jay stayed with me the whole time. He brought me snacks and he handed me honey-lemon drops so I didn't cough at a bad moment. The tattoo artist was pleased with the way it turned out. "I'll see you again in a couple of weeks for the color," he said.

I told Ford that the outline was done. He looked distracted. He said, "I have to make some calls to the East Coast this morning." Later, I walked into the surf shop. There was a strange mood in the shop. The guys were all talking about him. His friend said to me quietly, "He gave two weeks notice today; he's moving to Tahoe to be with her."

He never spoke to me again. I stopped looking for him when he arrived in the mornings; I avoided the street when the shop closed each evening. I kept going to my singing lessons. I clutched at every small hopeful sign in counseling with Jay. I got the tattoo colored in. It hurt a lot, and it took much longer to heal than the outline.

* * *

I was nervous on the drive to Kali's wedding. We played my CDs in the car; I tried to decide if I would really go through with it. At the wedding, Jay played acoustic guitar – "The Long and Winding

Road" – for the processional, my daughter was the flower girl, and my son, in his first navy blue jacket, was the ring boy. My heart was so full as I watched them all play their parts during the brief ceremony. Afterwards, we walked to the reception next door, and friends and family started giving toasts, passing a microphone from one to another. The groom's sisters stood up and welcomed Kali to the family as their new sister.

Suddenly I knew I wanted to sing – I took the microphone and stood up. I told the guests that I was taking voice lessons and I wanted their help to sing for the bride and groom. I taught them the chorus of "Darling Companion" and had them sing it with me once. And then I stepped into the body of the singer, just as I'd warmed up at every lesson. I sang, "Darling companion, Come on and give me understanding..." I got to the chorus, and waved to the guests to join me. The room swelled with voices, on key, off key, all together, "Oh oh oh oh, a little settling down with you is what she needs..." The singer in me finished the song alone, "...Love will always light our landing, I can depend on you!"

I ended, and handed off the microphone amidst laughter and applause. I sat back down at our table between Jay and my sister Jana. My daughter, who is incapable of tact, said, "Mommy, you weren't bad. You weren't really good either, but you weren't bad." That was high praise, but the very best part was seeing Jay and Jana stare at me with their mouths open. Jana said quietly to me, "We were so surprised, but we sang the chorus with you." Jay said, "You did fine. You brought us all along with you. I can't believe you did it."

* * *

175

The tattoo is gorgeous – it's centered on my lower back. With the color filled in, the tattoo comes to life, all greens, pinks and yellows. The sides of the tattoo are like vines, reaching out across my back. In the middle is the "Om" symbol, the Namaste. My yoga teacher leads us in a chant before and after each class: "The light that is in me recognizes and bows to the light that is in you. Namaste."

The tattoo curls across my skin. When I stand up, it's as if the tattoo is propelling me forward. I feel beautiful and courageous. This is real, this is who I am. I am being true to myself. Namaste.

Colleen Gregory (45) is a social worker living in Santa Cruz, California with her two lively children, three aloof cats, and one very understanding husband. She occasionally hosts mosaic workshops, works part-time counseling women and teens, and sings her heart out in the shower and other fine establishments.

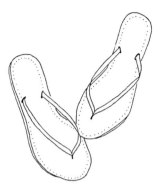

A Community to Call My Own

By Kim Merkin

When I first approached 40, I paused to look around me, and realized that the one gaping hole in my life was an absence of good friends. So, I did what comes naturally to me: I devised a zany way to create a new community. It was very me.

Well… Actually there are two me's. First, there is Me the super saleswoman. The always-on-call Me. The problem fixer. The merry patcher-up-of-things-about-to-go-wrong Me.

For the fifteen years leading up to 40, I had built a career in tradeshow exhibit sales. It's good money. It's exhilarating. And it's good money, if I forgot to mention that. I know people all over the world. I serve Fortune 100 clients. Fortune 500 clients. Fortune 1000 clients. I help start-ups you've never heard of display products as diverse as green olives and bra cups, shoulder pads and airport security luggage scanners. My exhibits are enormous, incredibly expensive portable "events," and I flit all over the mercantile world with them, to toy shows in Germany, machinery shows in Korea, electronics shows in Hong Kong, and a million and one times to Las Vegas, the glitzy trade show capital of the planet.

But there came this moment. It was just as I was comfortably moving through my late 30s. You may remember hearing about a little economic event called the dot.com crash. All those little Internet-based start-up companies – many of them my clients – who had been shoveling piles of cash at marketing events suddenly went Poof! And for an eerie moment or two, there was an unfamiliar silence in my busy little world. I found myself at home more. At home…there in the suburbs. Not in Las Vegas. Not in Paris. Not on an expense account. Not staying up 'til 2 a.m. partying with clients. Just a little bit of unfamiliar silence.

In that silence, I noticed that there were not a lot of people scurrying around me. I didn't like that. I had friends in New York. Friends in Germany. Friends in Ireland, for God's sake. But I didn't live in those places. Or more to the point, they didn't live next door to me. And I needed playmates.

Which is the other me. The fun-and-slightly-goofy-games Me. The Me who wants to plan an activity that we've never done before and go out and do it, no matter how people will react.

The only problem with this is… well…. It's kind of tough finding pals who are willing to be zany with me. On a business trip with creative types to Vegas, you can phone up someone's room and say, "Let's go see the drag queen show," and then hang out 'til all hours in the lounge drinking banana daiquiris or whatever. People on expense accounts do stuff like that. People in the suburbs, not so much. I needed entertainment. I needed fun people.

After a while, I started to get restless. I found that some of my oldest friends were at that nesting stage, spending more time at home with their young families. I wanted more friends in my life. My husband Kevin and I don't have children, so I couldn't tap into the mommy community. I don't officially have a religion, so I couldn't go trawling at local churches and synagogues for new buddies. I don't have any of those wholesome hobbies like Beanie Baby collecting, which might have allowed me to pop into the local Ramada Inn Convention Center on a Saturday morning to collect a posse of like-minded friends. I'm frequently out of town, so I never got into any fund-raising circles, political factions or social causes. My family and Kevin's live all over the country, so they aren't available on a daily basis. And as for Kevin, he has wonderful hobbies of his own. He's an avid biker and a marathon runner – both totally out of the question for me. Don't even bother suggesting it.

The realization was actually a little startling to me: I had built the strong pillars of a successful working world – connections, connections, connections. But at the threshold of 40, I had no community. As someone who placed a high premium on my business community, the realization that I lacked the same network in my personal life was a depressing notion.

So here is where the first Me kicked in – Me the problem-fixer.

Since I was trained from the working world to have goals, I set up a goal of having more friends. My goal: "Develop a circle of deeply satisfying friendships with women who live within 15 miles of my house." So okay, the 15 mile radius thing was a little arbitrary, but that's how I make attainable goals.

But how? Next step: "Devise a procedure for gathering this circle of women."

Do I go knocking on neighbors' doors? Should I begin introducing myself to the person standing in line next to me at the grocery store? I sought advice from the field. I surveyed as many friends and acquaintances as I could to ask them if they shared the same dilemma as I did.

As it turned out, I was far from alone in my desires. Far, far, far from alone. Every woman I queried immediately responded to my yearning for fellowship. I realized I was sparking something of a movement from all my surveying and questioning. A casually amassing association of local suburban women who wanted to be united in… in their desire to be united.

We christened our movement "EBUG" – the East Bay United Gals club. It was a corny moniker but it stuck. Our mission would be to create events with the sole purpose of giving a community of women an excuse to gather together. They would be women who live in the 925 or 510 area codes of the San Francisco Bay Area. And that was our entire charter.

The consensus probably wouldn't make sense to a political pollster, but the will of the club was that we wanted to meet new women, we wanted to spend more time getting to know our community, and we wanted to steer ourselves away from traditional groups and activities.

Our first event, in its entirety, consisted of four friends who each brought one other friend to a garden party. It was potluck and didn't cost anything. We held it at my landscapers' wonderfully over-the-top landscaped house in the Berkeley hills. Our group of eight sat in the garden surrounded by 10,000 plants, including ceramic bamboo shoots with penis tops. They were unusual landscapers, but this set the precedent for events that were safe and comfortable, yet just a bit left of center.

It went well. So for the next event, all eight women had to bring another new friend – taking us to sixteen women. We wouldn't double our membership at each meeting, but you get the idea, to bring in new faces and enjoy fun new activities.

Usually, the agenda is a theme potluck dinner at someone's house. Moving the event around helps us become better acquainted with our neighborhoods. "I've been in that house, and that house and that house," I can say as I drive through town. Among our themes, we've had a chocolate tasting, a hula-hoop lesson, and a book exchange (no actual reading of the book required). We have gone sailing, held a luau, made jewelry, enjoyed a spa/beauty night, and tattooed ourselves with henna. We also had a "Bring a covered dish and an unresolved personal problem" event. That meeting allowed us to air our favorite personal crises – not so much to fix or make them go away, but more to have a room full of sympathetic club members give each other a shoulder to cry on.

With another event – our "100 things we wanted to do in life" party – we actually attracted national attention. The *New York Times* asked if it could send a photographer to shoot the event. "Sure," we thought. "Why not?" Five of us appeared in a large photo in a *Sunday Times* feature about women and their new approaches to associations.

The idea of that particular evening was just to share our various unique dreams for ourselves. We each read ten items on our list. One woman shared that she wanted friends from three different generations. Another wanted to experience a Brazilian wax. Another wanted to fall in love again – regardless of whether it was with her husband. The candid responses were fascinating and bonding as a group. It was a powerful way to get to know one another.

Which is exactly what I hoped we would become as a club – a community of like-minded friends. After six years, EBUG is responsible for creating some of my closest personal friendships, and for strengthening my relationships with existing friends. Having this circle has made my life as a 40-something woman more peaceful and contented. With a community of friends, I don't feel pressure to prove anything to myself or my peers. I'm more comfortable in my own skin and I like my life. I know my career and how to do it well. I'm not trying to figure out what I'm good at any more. It's really a very freeing time.

The super-saleswoman Me still thrives. I still hop here and there with clients. But I am treating the fun-and-slightly-goofy-games Me with equal respect. Today, I would much rather share stories about our group than about my professional world, which dominated so much of my 20s and 30s. I've discovered that there are others out there just like me. And my club is a way to reach out and welcome them in. If I seem to connect with a woman about my age who lives in my area, I now have a conversation starting point: "Do you want to come to an EBUG event?"

And more often than not, she does.

———————

Kim Merkin (44) has been a trade show exhibit sales person for the last 20 years. She considers herself a glorified "carney" who, fortunately, makes a significantly better income and has a full set of teeth. She enjoys hiking the hills of Northern California, playing with her Tibetan Terrier, Bobbi, and hula-hooping. As a result of EBUG, she has united with over 150 cool gals – a community she's very proud to call her own.

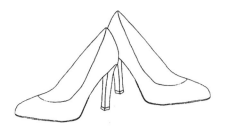

Sliding Away

By Regina Sewell

hrough the phone line that connects us, her voice sounds flat, dull. It's lost the luster and vibrancy that it had only a year ago. Her words come out slurred, as if the effort of talking is exhausting. I called her the day before yesterday to find out how her trip to Savannah, Georgia went, hoping to hear her usual excitement as she relived the trip with me over the phone. She couldn't remember any of the details. I'd hoped that today would be better, but she can't even remember that we talked two days ago. My heart feels like it's imploding. I want to reach back in time, back to the mother that remembered things, back to the mother who loved to travel and tell me every excruciating detail of her trip, back to the mother whose voice sounded vibrant and alive. I don't ask about Savannah.

Instead, I ask her about the cards she's making. We talk about the stamps she's using and how the new brand of pencils she bought are smoother and easier to use. I used to drift into boredom when she talked about making her cards. Now I'm asking questions about the stamps and pencils she's using. I'm grasping for connection.

We move on to the weather. It's warm and sunny in San Antonio. It's cold and rainy in Ohio. We both hate rain and cold weather. She tells me that she wishes I'd move back to Texas. Even in the flatness of her voice, I hear her longing and feel her pull. In this moment, I want nothing more than to go home, to hold her. I tell her that I wish I could go home too.

She starts to tell me about a teaching job she heard about, one that I have a good shot of getting because she knows the person who retired. I try to feel her love when she says this, but I start to panic at the thought of moving back to Texas.

I can't move back. It would be too painful. I cut her off. I have *chosen* to live far away from her. The naked truth of this choice hits me like a lead pipe. My inner critic begins to sneer, "Not only are you not *normal*, you're not even a good enough daughter to move back home to take care of your mother." My guilt sinks to shame.

The feeling rises up my spine and tightens around my throat. I don't know how to talk to her. I am afraid that she'll feel bad if I tell her how guilty and ashamed I feel. This leads to even more shame because I realize that I'd rather snap at her than let her see my vulnerability, and sit with her in hers.

I take a deep breath and gather up my courage. Fumbling for words, I apologize for snapping at her. Before she can respond, I admit for the first time that I'm afraid that I'll be shunned or beaten for being a lesbian if I move back to Texas. We don't usually talk much about my sexual orientation so this admission feels scary. Tears stream down my cheeks as I talk. I hear myself pleading with her to understand why I can't move home and to love me anyway. I desperately want her to hear that I'm not rejecting her. And I want reassurance that she doesn't reject me either. But my desperation feels too raw. She doesn't say anything. The silence is terrifying.

I want to tell her that I'm afraid of losing her. I want to ask her what it's like to not remember. But I don't think that either of us can handle that level of truth, so I say nothing. One of us changes the subject, away from the heart and back to the safety of details. She tells me about the cards she's made again and that she wishes I were there. I say goodbye, knowing that she probably won't remember this conversation either.

When I hang up, I'm able to distance myself from my immediate pain and feel the weight of the realization that the mother I knew is gone. I'd seen the signs of her mental deterioration on my last visit home a year before, but I'd denied their significance. We'd gotten lost on the way to the library. When she realized that she had no idea where the library was, she'd slipped into despair. It was like watching someone who's lost a limb finally realize that their limb is not there anymore, that it's gone for good. Even though I sensed that her memory was sliding away, I convinced myself that we could fix the problem. Unfortunately, there aren't prosthetics for your mind or wheelchairs for your memory. When it goes, it's gone. Not even the Alzheimer's drugs like Aricept and Namenda can bring back the memory. At best, they forestall some of the symptoms. Stripped of my hope, I don't remember when I've felt so alone.

I only have one friend who understands what I'm going through, and her answering machine tells me, "I'm sorry that I'm not available to take your call right now." She lives thousands of miles away, so the hug I need would be a bit of a challenge anyway. My other friends simply don't understand. When I told them that my mother forgot my birthday for the first time last year, they cut me off and wished me a happy birthday. When I tried to explain how significant this was, they said things like, "Well, she *is* old..."

I don't share my grief about my mother's slipping memory because to do so would leave me feeling emotionally naked. I'd be devastated if anyone I confided in misunderstood or dismissed my pain. I've never been much of a risk taker, so I mask my tears with laughter. I joke that because my mother's short term memory is shot, talking to her is like talking to someone who's high on pot. I turn getting lost into a stand-up routine (in my full-blown Texas accent): "So we're drivin' down this road and all the sudden, it just stops, like they ran out of money or somethin'. There aren't even cows around to ask directions from. So we try to figure out what direction we're goin' from the shadows...."

Perhaps this raw vulnerability is why other people who are watching their parents drift off into the fog of dementia and Alzheimer's don't really share their pain either. And because they don't share their experience, we as a culture tend to minimize their pain. It's much easier to discount someone's pain than to feel the vulnerability of the human condition. I still remember the sense of indignant frustration I felt with a friend of mine for not setting boundaries with his mother. She called him several times a day to talk about news shows on PBS, and to complain about the particular recordings the local classical music station chose to play. He talked to her at least once a day even when we were on vacation. When she ran out of bananas and we had to come home several days early, I wanted to strangle him. She lived within easy walking distance of two grocery stores, couldn't she just get her own damned bananas? And even if she couldn't walk to the store, couldn't he have a neighbor or a friend drop them off? I'm sure he picked up on my feelings. I didn't understand then that he was racing against time.

I suppose that on some level, my pain feels too complicated and too raw to express to my friends. To really reach out to them would require me to admit, in public, that for all these years that I've supposedly been "grown-up," I've been clinging to the dream that someday, my mother could fix my broken heart. I'd have to acknowledge the fact that there is a part of me that holds on to the belief that someday she will wrap me in her arms like a little child, and all the sorrow and fear that I've been carrying around since childhood would ebb away.

I was sexually abused as a child so I've always felt like I was somehow dirty, rotten or just plain bad. The only way to be lovable, my child self reasoned, was to say or do the right thing, to find that magic key that would make it possible for my mother to love me unconditionally. Perhaps things would have been different if my mother had protected me from my grandfather, but she didn't. I don't think she knew. I don't think that she could know.

I'd also have to admit that I am still not taking responsibility for my own happiness because I've been desperately waiting all my life for her to prove to me that she loves me so that I could, perhaps, love myself. I've heard it said that the longest journey is from the head to the heart. For years, I've known, with my head, that my mother couldn't heal my childhood wounds. The silver lining of watching my mother slide into dementia is that in my heart, I finally understand this.

I'm finally taking responsibility for my own healing. Instead of wishing that my mother would heal my childhood wounds, I take time out to visualize my adult self nurturing and comforting that poor mixed up little kid who thinks she's so unlovable. I'm finally starting to become the mother to myself that I've always wanted.

Regina Sewell (43) has a Ph.D. in Sociology and an M.Ed. in Community Counseling. She teaches Sociology at Ohio State University and has a private practice in counseling in Worthington, Ohio. When not working, she can be found dancing to live music, playing guitar with friends and strangers, splashing in the waves of whatever beach she's landed on, and tearing up the asphalt (or at least going as fast as she can peddle) on her Dolci Elite road bike. She is the author of "We're Here! We're Queer! Get Used to Us! Survival Skills for a Hostile World." Her bi-weekly column, "Insight Out," can be found in Columbus Outlook Weekly.

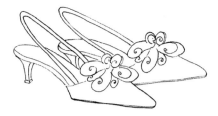

Tangled Up with Two

By Ona Gritz

Sometime during the angst-ridden year I was fourteen, or maybe it was the angst-ridden year I was fifteen, my mother told me she didn't have any confidence in herself until she turned forty.

The statement was interesting enough to pull me out of my self-absorption for a moment.

"What happened when you were forty?"

But as usual, she was elusive. She shrugged, saying, "Nothing. I just saw things differently," and went off to start dinner. I sat on the sticky vinyl couch, the pages of my unfinished homework spread out on a small metal folding table in front of me, wondering.

My mother died six months before my fortieth birthday, so she didn't get to see that it happened to me too, this unexpected late blossoming and new self-assurance. Nor would she know of the resulting craziness I found myself in during my forty-second year, caught in a tangle of lovers I only dreamt about in my twenties.

To be fair, things had begun to improve when, a few years earlier, my handsome, overbearing husband decided to leave me. For him it was a whim, a decision made during finals week in graduate school on a caffeine drenched all-nighter. He never intended to be held to it.

But within weeks of his departure, I realized I felt light, unburdened. Our son, Ethan, was three at the time, and irrationally in love with me. We became groupies on the children's music circuit that summer, eating our dinners on our laps while Tom Chapin or Raffi serenaded us with songs the two of us had come to know by heart.

I didn't think about dating that first year, but when spring rolled around a second time with its elongated days and irrepressible birdsong, I suddenly felt a need that not even the most rocking rendition of *Skip to My Lou* could fill.

I was thirty-eight, flushed, I think now, with the first hints of that confident glow that would mark my forties. At an art opening held, oddly enough, in a small women's clothing store, I met a guy.

Paul wasn't nearly as cute as my ex, but he had a kind face and was warm and funny. And, as I found out the very next night, he was hotter in bed at fifty than my ex had been at twenty-one. We started sleeping together a couple of nights a week, Paul lightly ringing my buzzer after Ethan was certain to be deeply asleep. By then, what little confidence I'd had had been rubbed away by a husband who rarely looked at me, and even more rarely touched me. But now Paul, a figure painter who spent many of his working hours with gorgeous nude and scantily clad models, ran his discerning fingers over my body and told me I was beautiful. Slowly, tentatively, I started to believe him.

Paul and I also went out on dates. They were the kind of dates I rarely had in my twenties when, like most of my girlfriends, I had guy friends I either slept with or didn't. My ex-husband was different from the others in that he called me his girlfriend; but our actual dates dwindled down to pizza and videos at home within two months of our knowing each other.

I suppose, by comparison, Paul was old-fashioned. He loved to get dressed up and go out to nice restaurants. He held my hand in movie theaters. I imagine he'd have opened car doors for me too, had I thought to wait.

I felt coddled and adored. And when, a year into our courtship, my parents took ill and died within months of each other, I clung to him.

He moved in with us. Paul didn't want to take on a step-parenting role with Ethan, but he was kind to him and good at taking care of me. He enjoyed fixing things around the house. He did all the driving and many of the domestic errands. In those ways, he was much like my father. In fact, I'd given him my father's leather jacket which still bore a lingering scent of Old Spice. Sometimes, I'd bury my nose in his shoulder to recall the feeling of being someone's daughter again.

Paul continued to tell me I was beautiful and, for the first time in my life, I walked around as a beautiful woman does: back straight and head up high, glinting eyes and a slightly knowing smile. Men frequently smiled back. I imagined telling my mother that I too learned to love myself in my forties.

I felt happy, though slightly restless. Another characteristic Paul shared with my father was a complete lack of interest in books. I'm an author and a librarian. On quiet evenings at home, my favorite companion is a well-written novel. Paul flipped through art magazines. He kept a book on wine tasting in the bathroom. But just as my father had, every evening when he was ready to relax, Paul turned on the television.

No matter. I had women friends who shared my taste in fiction, loved to talk about what they were reading, and made wonderful recommendations. And while I felt there was a large part of me that Paul would never understand, I took comfort in the words of a favorite poet, Stephen Dunn, who wrote of relationships: "it's doubtful she will be enough for you/or you for her. You must have friends/of both sexes. When you get together/ you must feel everyone has brought/his fierce privacy with him/and is ready to share it…"

Paul was good at sharing his private self with me. He also gave me a safe place in which to share my own. But when the part I wanted to share had to do with my intellectual life, Paul, more often than not, literally fell asleep.

On my forty-first birthday I had what I thought of not as a midlife crisis, but rather, a midlife epiphany. My mother had died at eighty-two, and it struck me that, for all I knew, I might be at the exact midpoint of my own life. Was I doing all that I could to lead the fullest life possible? What, if anything, was lacking? The answer I came to was that I wasn't writing enough. It was my truest passion, yet I squeezed it in instead of making it a real priority.

I went back to writing poetry, my first love, when I realized that one of the reasons I didn't write regularly was that I was waiting for uninterrupted chunks of time in which to work on large projects. Poetry would be a better fit during my parenting years. I formed a critique circle with two women poets who also accompanied me to occasional readings. Yet as I began to write more seriously, I found myself craving professional feedback and a larger literary community. When I discovered that Stephen Dunn was teaching a weekend workshop nearby, I quickly signed up.

I found Stephen to be an inspiring and supportive teacher. He praised my poems in a way other students said was rare for him. I came away feeling encouraged about my work and charged by the richness of a weekend spent with other writers. But that's not the whole story. I also came away with a crush on one of the other students.

Dan was a good poet with a sweet, attentive disposition. We sat next to each other in Stephen's workshop, and I loved the gentle but precise suggestions he gave to our classmates. Though we didn't talk much during that busy weekend, I could tell he was drawn to me. When he asked for my email address on the last day, I thought of the line in Stephen's poem that implied that having friends of both sexes was good for a relationship.

"Take my phone number too," I said.

The night that Dan called, Paul had fallen asleep, as he often did, in front of the television. Dan and I talked for four hours. It was a remarkable conversation that flowed from writing to relationships to childhood memories and back again with an ease that was new to both of us. By the time we hung up, I had the sinking feeling that my relationship with Paul was in serious trouble. At the same time, I felt elated.

Dan and I tried to keep our relationship platonic for awhile, but our attraction to each other was hard to ignore. We continued to have long, late night conversations, during which we often read to each other – usually poems, sometimes rather steamy poems, though we pretended to have picked them solely for their literary merit. We also signed up for a workshop with the poet Molly Peacock that met on four consecutive Sundays. I feigned surprise at the coincidence that we both wanted to take her class.

On the fourth Sunday of Molly's workshop, we found ourselves making out like teenagers in a café. After a few guilt-ridden days, I confessed to Paul. I wasn't entirely surprised when he suggested we try an open relationship. After all, monogamy was something I had prized and to which he had more or less relented.

"Have whatever physical relationship you want," he told me. "Just don't give him your heart."

The comment frightened me, in part because I was looking for him to set a boundary I wasn't able to set for myself, but mostly because it told me how little Paul understood me. Did he really think my body would be tempted elsewhere if my heart hadn't already led the way?

And so, at the age of forty-two, I became a woman with two lovers. Had you told me this would have happened twenty years prior, I'd have been astonished. Yet I imagine I would have been cheering my older self on. But then, at twenty-two, I didn't have a household to consider breaking up, or a child whose feelings were a deep concern. Nor did I have a set of values already in place that I thought of as unshakeable. It would have been the perfect time to have two sweet, caring men in love with me. But, alas, like my mother, I was a late bloomer. And while I might have been ecstatic to find myself in this position back then, I now found it excruciating.

My experiment with polygamy only lasted a few months. While neither of my lovers pressured me, I knew for myself that I had to make a decision.

In the end, I left Paul. In a number of ways, it was the harder choice. We had a loving relationship. Ethan was comfortable with our shared domestic life. I felt emotionally safe and cared for in our home. Also, there were things about Dan I couldn't yet know. With him, I'd really be starting at the beginning.

In truth, the two men have a number of qualities in common. They're both gentle, affectionate, and openly emotional. Dan's intellectual curiosity and love of literature certainly swayed me. Our lovemaking also proved to be a deeper, more connected experience. But if I had to boil it down, I'd say it was conversation that ultimately won me over.

Back when Paul first told me to have whatever physical relationship I wanted with Dan, he also said, "Just don't tell me anything." So instead I talked to Dan as I struggled with this unexpected balancing act. He let me cry and name my fears. Together, we imagined different scenarios, until I figured out what I most wanted in a partner, which, in the end, proved to be someone I could show myself to completely. A lover and a confidante in the same person – something I didn't know was possible until, in mid-life, I realized I was lucky enough to have found it.

———

Ona Gritz (45) is a writer, librarian and single mother. She performs this juggling act in Hoboken, NJ, birthplace of baseball and Frank Sinatra, and home to a stellar view of the Manhattan skyline. Ona is a great shower singer and a terrible guitarist. She does a mean Roger Daltrey imitation on the rare occasions her son woos her into playing *Rock Band*. Ona writes a monthly column for the online journal, *Literary Mama*. She is also a prize-winning poet and the author of two children's books. Her essays have been published in numerous journals and anthologies. In 2007, she received two Pushcart nominations.

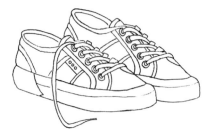

Stumbling into Cyberspace

By Amy Kossoff Smith

*M*y fingers raced across the keyboard, and my heart pounded as I heard the school bus wheels screech to a halt outside our house. Only a few more precious minutes to get that last e-mail out before the kids would bound through the door, kick off their shoes, throw their backpacks in the hall and demand a snack.

It was time to shift gears from work to kids, knowing full well that while my second shift was just starting, the third one (post-bedtime work catch-up) still lay ahead. After years of balancing three kids with my home-based PR business, I had added a scrumptious new project to my already-full plate. I started a website and blog that combined my organizational skills, my writing and PR background, and my passion for motherhood.

This latest entrepreneurial fire was ignited when I turned 40. For my birthday I went with some girlfriends to a spa where I paused for that rare moment of reflection in an otherwise activity-driven life. The lycra-clad fitness instructor had us lying on mats: "Breathe in. Breathe out. Breathe in. Breathe out." As desperate as I was for a true break, I was having trouble following her instructions to "clear my mind." I found my mind wandering to my lengthy to-do list and unanswered e-mails. So much to do....No, no, no...breathe in, breathe out. As I struggled to clear my mind, it hit me that I'd spent most of my professional and personal life focused on other people's needs. Helping to fulfill other peoples' dreams.

But as I lay there on that mat trying to breathe, the writer in me decided that 40 needed to be *my* chapter. I realized that it was time to pursue a personal dream of my own that could bring more passion, fun, and enjoyment to my career. As a journalist, I'd written articles for newspapers and magazines; as a publicist, I'd pitched press releases and managed countless special events. But one journalistic feat that I had yet to accomplish, but had always yearned for, was to write a book about something I really cared about, something to showcase my own magic tricks for managing the hardest job in my life: motherhood. Soon I began walking into bookstores, eyeing the packed shelves like valuable real estate, wondering if and when I could earn a spot.

As a working mom, I had constantly found my business world and personal world colliding. Over the years, I had naturally begun to use my work tools to organize our home life. Complicated carpools? No problem, a color-coded spreadsheet will do the trick. Painting estimates? Make sure you ask each person the same five questions – display the answers on a chart. Chores for the kids? Lay it out so all can see. Chart after chart, spreadsheet after spreadsheet, my business skills were guiding me through motherhood, providing me with much valued order in my home. Though I knew that this approach might not be the answer for everyone, I had been asked for help from enough other busy moms to know that I had tools other people could use. So with a computer full of spreadsheets, checklists and essays, I revisited my idea from years ago, an idea that had lain dormant since the birth of my third son five years ago. I decided to write the book on which I'd based my adult family life, The Business of Motherhood.

Tenacious, I immediately wrote a proposal, called agents and set up meetings. I was told that first I would need a website and blog. My reaction was measurable and fortunately silent. "What *is* a blog? What have I missed here?" I thought. I felt completely deflated.

The social marketing world was completely foreign to me. Even my young kids seemed more savvy at downloading videos, text messaging, and Internet research than I. But removed as I felt from this virtual universe, I was motivated and determined to join, both to communicate my message as well as to understand this world my kids were entering.

I knew that the investment of time, energy, and money in this venture would be significant and I couldn't see any income generation in the first phase (or second or third). I started to question my plans. Could I throw one more ball in the air, already juggling so much between work and home? Should I divert energy from my PR firm, my consistent bread and butter, to start what could be no more than a hobby that would suck time, energy, and money from our family bank account?

Forty hit me the same year my youngest stepped on the kindergarten bus. With him in school, I had planned to use any spare time to go through the stacks and envelopes of family photos that I needed to put into albums, volunteer more at all three of my boys' classrooms, and perhaps even have some unscheduled time for me. Breathe in, breathe out.

Instead, I found myself uncontrollably driven to start this new venture. I felt an intense desire, like nothing I'd felt in a long time, to go out on a limb, take a personal risk, and be comfortable with success or failure.

So, leveraging technology I didn't even know existed, I found myself creating a blog, then a website, while at the same time fueling my passion for writing. My coaches: professionals who were half my age. Even those a quarter of my age knew more than I did at first.

"Mom, aren't you a little *old* for Facebook?" my 10-year-old asked. Little did he know that I would soon be ten steps ahead of him. If nothing else.

At worst, I was keeping up with the technology that defined my children's universe, and, at best, I was embarking on a mission to help other mothers.

I felt my journalism skills kick into high gear: writing, researching, links, statistics tracking, subscriptions, animated headlines, graphics research – it started fitting together like pieces in a puzzle. Finally, my first website was complete – I couldn't believe the functionality that we were able to build into it.

"You did a great job, and I really appreciate all you did to go outside the box and make this what it is," I told the designer. "I hope this site is something you'll be proud of, because I certainly am."

"Yeah, uh, thanks…" the web designer muttered humbly over the phone.

"I have one final question, and I hope this won't offend you in any way," I started. "How old are you?" He sounded so young, and having never met in person, I honestly had no idea.

"I'm 19."

"You're 19!?" I was sure I'd heard something wrong, but he couldn't have said 90. Suddenly, it all clicked. The lingo, the laid back attitude, and quite frankly, the key to technology he gave me.

He was half my age and young enough to be my son, and he was one of the best teachers I'd ever had.

So we built it. I built it. But would anyone come? I felt like I'd cooked my best meal, put on my favorite party dress, and was waiting for the doorbell to ring. And ring it did…

I remember the first time I went to the visitor map, an online traffic counter with a map of the world displaying flags in each country where an "eyeball" had visited my site.

I shrieked.

"Mommy, what's wrong?" asked my son, running into my office.

I was staring at the computer screen, flags popping up on the world map, one by one as the page loaded, showing visitor traffic to the site. Pop, pop, pop.

"Nothing, sweetie, everything's okay, but someone just looked at my site from China! And England! And Iraq!"

I hadn't even started my press campaign yet. So apparently the announcement I had sent to 160 friends and family was actually making its way around the world. It reminded me of an old shampoo commercial, "And she told two friends…and she told two friends… and so on, and so on." I was awed by the simplicity and the sheer power of word of mouth – thousands and thousands of visitors in the first few weeks alone. I had read about the power of these new marketing tools, but now I was experiencing them for myself firsthand. I realized I was part of the "older generation" now, but I was catching up and would not be left behind. Technology was going to transform my dream into reality. It was going to connect me with women around the world.

I'll never forget my first interview on FOX News. I was used to putting clients on TV and convincing nervous interviewees that it was really simple, that they shouldn't be nervous. Now that *I* would be the one in front of the camera, I felt my heart racing, my palms sweating, my teeth clenching. I woke up every two hours the night before, paranoid that the alarm wouldn't go off.

But it did…and the lack of sleep probably slowed me down a bit on air, which was good. My message – how to save time and money for moms – flowed naturally. Other than an unknown, very errant strand of hair in my face (despite a very long session with assorted gels, sprays, and my hairdryer), I made it through, and skipped to my car like a school girl just asked to the big dance.

And what a dance it is! I've met Mompreneurs from around the world, online and in person. I have shared the thrill of new ventures and the power of collaborative marketing like I've never experienced before. From a former TV reporter turned blogger/fiction novelist in my own home town to a nutritionist from Sydney, Australia, my network expands daily.

I feel new self-confidence and comfort in the technology that truly petrified me a year ago. These tools are like building blocks in my hi-tech playroom. I've become enthralled with the endless options that are only a click away, adding form and function to my websites. I find myself urging others to pursue the Cyberpath that has given me such incredible fulfillment in such a short period of time. I feel like I am learning, growing and serving in a way that feels wonderfully energizing. I am struck by what a difference a year can make, and am now wondering what next year will bring. Maybe I'll even finally make time for those family photo albums.

Amy Kossoff Smith (41) is married in Maryland with three boys under the age of 11. She founded BusinessofMotherhood.com, a site that presents motherhood as a legitimate and valuable job, and provides tips and tactics to help moms manage their busy lives. Her blog has regular posts about topics of interest to the business of motherhood. An internationally recognized Mompreneur, she is a McClatchy-Tribune Wire columnist, with weekly columns appearing in newspapers and online nationwide. She runs Write Ideas, Inc., a public relations and promotions firm she founded in 1992. When she's not working, she relishes a sweaty "Body Pump" class where breathing is mandatory.

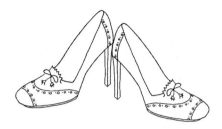

Getting My Mother Sober

By Erin St. John Kelly

ate in the afternoon of Easter Sunday last year, my mother arrived at my house for dinner holding on hard to my stepfather's arm, sporting a fresh, scabby shiner. She'd managed to fall *up* the stairs, slamming into the baluster of her staircase the night before. I nudged her towards a chair in my little kitchen as efficiently and as subtly as I could, hoping to minimize her mobility and the possibility of another accident.

My mother sat at the head of the table, having a slur of a rant to no one in particular. Among my assembled guests of friends and family, one of my sisters and her daughter sat quietly leaking tears at their places. My eldest daughter left the table after a short while and the rest of the children followed her. Their grandmother was scaring them during the appetizer course and they opted for crackers and cheese in the next room instead. She was impenetrable, only vaguely resembling the person they'd known as their grandmother. The adults knew the reason, but the kids didn't.

My brother James had died earlier that year. It was sudden, out of the blue, and far, far away from my mother's bucolic college town. She hadn't been able to say goodbye. She hadn't seen his body. The night he died she lamented that she never should have let him go. As if he'd asked, and as if he would have obeyed the demand she never made. She couldn't relate to the distant place he'd died except through the story of "Butch Cassidy and the Sundance Kid" because they too had died in Tupiza, Bolivia. James wasn't robbing banks and he didn't die in a shoot-out. He and his wife were backpacking around the world, doing good works, before they settled down to raise a family. He died of altitude sickness in an Andean emergency room that had no oxygen mask. He came home as a box of ashes.

My mother was raised on a farm, the middle child of seven girls. She was the first ever in her family to go to college. She survived a bout with breast cancer, a stint in women's prison for civil disobedience, and Woodstock in the rain. My mother was already a functional drunk, but it was her despair from James' death that triggered her descent into raging alcoholism.

My mother was so drunk she smelled. She wore the same sweat pants and sweat shirt day in and day out. She had once loved a martini – we called them garbage-tinis because she'd pretend it was good for her by adorning it with limp, brown vegetables culled from the drawers of the fridge, creating a stinky salad in a fancy glass. Now she was pared down to gin in a coffee mug while lying in bed.

My mother has read all of Proust. She has probably spent more time immersed in the matters of Congress (via C-SPAN) than have most actual members. As a matter of course, three televisions and at least one radio were on at all times, and two or three daily newspapers were ingested. When we were growing up she took us to rock concerts, peace rallies and hitchhiking through the Yukon. Then, a loud slide into nothing. The televisions were all on but she didn't know what was happening on them. She didn't know what time of day it was, light or dark – it was irrelevant. She was either in a rage, or on the verge of one. She complained that she didn't hear from us, her children, enough. We did call, but she didn't remember having spoken to us. One winter afternoon at my mother's house, my eight-year-old daughter realized that my mother was surprised to see her every time she walked past. She said to me, "Mom, I am worried about Granny's memory." I explained that Granny was really sad about James and drank too much alcohol in an effort to feel better.

My five remaining siblings and I felt helpless for more than a year to address her drinking, except among each other. His death brought the revelation that the family had depended on James, the middle child, to be our emotional and cultural center. Now we had lost him. He was so steadfast, earnest and good. He signed off all his emails from abroad with this Mark Twain quote: "Travel is fatal to prejudice, bigotry, and narrow-mindedness, and many of our people need it sorely on these accounts. Broad, wholesome, charitable views of men and things cannot be acquired by vegetating in one little corner of the earth all one's lifetime."

James was also a worrier. Be it concern for the global state of humanity or trying to eat healthier, he was on it. And he had helped me deal with Mom. No one hated my mother's drinking like James had.

I hadn't planned to confront Mom for everyone's Easter dinner. I had planned to serve a specially ordered ham instead. I had been rolling around the need to deal with her in my mind, but hadn't been able to form a real plan of how and when to do it. There's no good time for an intervention with your mother.

It started by accident. I sat next to her and suggested she eat something every now and again, maybe even drink a glass of water. I offered to get her one. She mumbled that she couldn't, that I just didn't understand how it felt to be her. She dropped the sickening bomb I knew she had, but didn't think I had it in me to withstand. She didn't save it up. It came out fast. "You haven't lost a child," she moaned. Everything froze. All the chopping, washing, table-setting and chat ceased.

My voice shook and I paused. Then I continued, motivated by the eternal regret and sorrow that I'd experience if I just let her die without trying to make her stop. I had to feel like I tried.

"You haven't lost a child." It was what I feared she would say. I felt almost guilty for not having a dead child myself. That without one, I had no understanding and therefore no grounds to complain. "No, I haven't," I said. Then it came to me why I could confront her. "But I have lost a brother. And now I am losing my mother. And my children are losing their grandmother." There was more that just tumbled out, but I can no longer remember what else I said. My mother sat quietly waiting for me to finish. "Well, dear, Mommy loves you very much, but now she has to go," she said, as she put her hand on my shoulder to raise herself up from the table. My stepfather came around to get her, led her out the front door, put her in the car and they drove out into the snowy night.

I know that it is completely irrational to feel like James' death was a personal failure of mine, but there it is. I did. As the oldest child I had always felt a conflicted mix of power and responsibility. I fixed things. I adjudicated. I felt I had failed everyone by not bringing him back from Bolivia alive. At the funeral home in La Paz, I saw him for the last time through the glass window of a little blue coffin. His shoulders were cramped against the wooden walls of a box built for a small Andean native – the biggest coffin his wife was able to find. I am haunted by his face with his lips pursed in the way they looked before he was going to say something that mattered to him. He hated Mom's drinking. I couldn't be so weak as to fail him and the family by letting Mom die a drunk.

Back in New York and at my desk on Monday I wrote my mother an email to restate in print what I'd said at Easter dinner – I was afraid that my spoken words wouldn't stick. I didn't know how else to try to get through. I hoped that she would be able to process it, staring at the screen in her own time. In my email I begged her to stop, to take some pity on us – the survivors – her children and her grandchildren. Must we watch her kill herself? And then I typed what I had been unable to say: was the death of one of us worth more than the other five of us alive?

I sent a copy of my email to my siblings right after sending it to my mother. I didn't want her to feel ambushed so I didn't cc them. But I wanted them to be aware of what I'd done, the possible horrors I'd unleashed. I waited with a panicky, shiny sense of dread for reaction – from them and from her.

On Wednesday, I was sitting at my desk when an email gently floated across my computer desktop that simply said, "You're right.

209

I quit." Oh my God, it's a suicide note I thought, and I dialed the phone, to see if I could stop her or if it was too late. There she was on the other end of the phone. I was at work so I couldn't say much except "Really? What can I do to help?"

My husband and I scrambled to find her a place and the funds to get her into rehab. We enlisted my baby sister (with those special youngest child powers) to try to convince her to go somewhere to dry out. I feared she would experience the sweating kind of DTs with hallucinations and bugs crawling the walls. "Let me try it my way," my mother said to her, "If that doesn't work then I promise to do it your way," she said. She and my stepfather joined AA.

It's been more than a year. She showers. She drinks seltzer and fruit juice spritzers in wine glasses. She goes to weekly AA meetings. A former reporter, she listens intently to other people's tales of horror and redemption. And she thanks me all the time for writing the note. "I want to be sober until the day that I die," she announced last summer. I believe her. My mother is nothing if not a zealous participator, a whole-hearted committer to things. She's recommenced being her old quirky self, protesting for peace in front of the post office, glutting herself on news and stuffing her grandchildren full of snacks.

And now, even her sense of humor is reviving. On Mother's Day this year she took me and two of my sisters out for dinner. She explained it was to make up for whatever she'd done wrong during our entire lives. She was practicing an AA step, and we had about an hour. We sipped delicious, unembellished tap water and I asked her what the secret element to her resolve was. "Maternal instinct," she said, "I don't want to worry the children. It's not the way it's supposed to be."

Erin St. John Kelly (45) is the eldest of the eight children from her parents' many marriages. She and her husband have two daughters. Being a sister, daughter or wife is much more complicated than being a mother, which has surprised her with its greatness. She has lived in Brooklyn, New York for almost 20 years excepting brief sojourns to Brooklyn-like neighborhoods in Buffalo, New York and Chicago. She is a Canadian from Montreal, Quebec. She had a big party to celebrate turning 40 because she never had a prom and got married at City Hall. She's hoping she'll feel that good about turning 50. She has anxiety about all the reading she's not doing, but her mother assures her that when she's old, like her, she'll get to it. Writing she is most proud of has appeared in *The New York Times, Gourmet* Magazine, *Brain,Child* Magazine and on WBFO, the Buffalo NPR station.

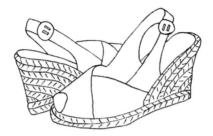

Good Enough

By Jennifer Lear

The underwater handstand contest nearly did me in. Until that moment, when I willed my lungs to push a few seconds beyond comfort, water had always soothed me by stilling my breath, my thoughts, my sense of time. Chalk it up to being born under an Aquarius astrological sign or to spending childhood summers with a chlorine-faded, Stars 'n Stripes Speedo as my uniform, but floating has always been my preferred method of self-medicating. In fact, if my Ob/Gyn had offered underwater births, I would have dived right in.

But while trying to outlast my daughters' handstands in the hotel pool a few months after turning 40, I found myself in the grip of a terror I had never before experienced in the water. Instead of floating in a soothing and meditative state of suspension, I felt seized. Totally stopped. My heart nearly stopped, my breathing nearly stopped, my control nearly stopped – everything stopped while I was held prisoner within the crushing walls of water closing in on me, suffocating thoughts tearing through my mind. I tried to push those thoughts away and restore my sense of serenity, but nothing I did could calm me.

Days before, I learned that my college friend, Kate, had drowned in her home after a torrent of rainwater broke through the foundation, trapping her inside a basement recording studio. The news unhinged me. It was too random, too insane, too violent to be real. I could wrap my brain around heart attacks, cancer, car accidents . . . but this, so stunning and incomprehensible; it was the stuff of nightmares, not reality. Holding my breath as I balanced upside down in the water that had always buoyed and restored me, I found it impossible to wash away the image of Kate's last moments.

Kate with the lithe limbs and the fly-girl dance moves. Kate, whose uninhibited cartoon laugh rivaled Betty Rubble's, but whose silky, sultry voice evoked Lauren Bacall. Kate the storyteller who could have the entire room under her spell whether narrating "A Tree Grows in Brooklyn" or musing about her day. Kate, who at 20 was more settled in her unique skin than most of us are decades later. Perhaps because she seemed to have had this head start, she crammed a lot into the decades between 20 and 40 – becoming the Meryl Streep of the audio-book world, using her distinctive voice to bring characters alive in award-winning recordings. Kate's stunning accomplishments and her premature death left me wondering, "Am I living big enough?"

As I reflected on how I'd spent the last 20 years, it seemed my life was an odd mix of impossible self-demands tempered with worry that each success increased the odds of a commensurate and compensating catastrophe. Rather than contenting in my blessings or good luck (and perhaps, in part, because I felt so blessed), I kept myself up at night dreading the illnesses, deaths, or other ordeals that would inevitably strike to even the score.

At first, Kate's death – the utter randomness of it – magnified these fears. I hoped her loss might be a catalyst, spurring me to begin my Broadway career, open a bakery, or become the next Oprah. But instead, it paralyzed me. If you can drown in your own home at 41, what's the point of any of this?

Something changed for me in the days after the underwater handstand contest. There was no defining moment, no flash of insight, but I began to see as liberating the randomness of my life that had always haunted me. Not in a "What I do doesn't make a damn bit of difference so why bother?" kind of way, but in a way that would please Anna Quindlen: "I show up, I listen, I try to laugh." And though I'm still not living big – I haven't done a fraction of the things I planned to do, hoped I would do, or still dream of doing – I now believe that what I've done is good enough.

Maybe I'd feel differently if I'd ever faced a true hardship, but I've been blessed with 40 years in which nothing awful has happened. I've always had loving family and friends, including a husband who thinks I'm getting better with age; a safe home; good health; and more than my fair share of joy, money, and food (let's hope the killer metabolism lasts another 40 years). There was some nasty acne during law school, a hernia operation, one breast cancer scare, and a colossal brain freeze as a law firm associate (when a memo is stamped "PRIVILEGED AND CONFIDENTIAL" it's not a good idea to send it to opposing counsel). I'm not a Pollyanna, but really, what do I have to complain about?

And really, what did I ever have to complain about? Nothing substantial has changed in the last ten years of my life. I have the same sense of balance now that I've had for over a decade. The kids are out of diapers but aren't dating or driving. My days are a satisfying blend of family-time, friend-time, and me-time, which means never quite enough husband-time. I work, I travel, I volunteer a bit, and I veg out and slack off too. So why am I only now finding contentment? Maybe it's that 40 seems like the halfway point. Maybe I finally feel like I've spent enough time here to have made memories sufficient to live on after I'm gone. Kate had only 41 years, and even though we all wanted more time with her, those years were enough to keep her vivid in my soul for the rest of my days.

I'm convinced I've had enough time to touch those closest to me in the same way, and yet I can't even point to what it is I've done. There was no great American novel or invention, and the last award I won was Mrs. McDonnell's Meister Singer plaque in 6th grade. So even if it's not what the world would consider a Big Life – complete with a host of patents, positions, and papers designed to impress classmates at my 20th college reunion – I'm okay with it, and I'm not focusing on the what-ifs. I keep coming back to the little memories I've made with family and friends: climbing into the crib to snuggle with my children; singing for friends on a whim in a Barcelona restaurant; body-surfing with my husband down the face of Mt. Rainier, and filling my fruit-hating daughter's lunch bag with apples on April Fool's Day (I'm not *that* mean; I showed up later with the real lunch). Little memories just big enough and good enough for me.

I'm not sure why these recollections outweigh those I'm less proud of: never teaching my daughters to tie their shoes, subjecting them to ridicule for being the only middle-schoolers without cell phones (or breasts, as they keep reminding me), and that time I didn't speak up when the Post Office clerk gave me too much change. But somehow, the good outshines the bad.

And while it's true that it's easy to be content in these small pleasures and embrace life when it's as free of hardship as mine has been, I know that there are trials in store for me. I'm now trying to accept it without dreading it. I try not to pressure myself to squeeze as much as I can out of each moment of my day. I choose contentment over fear. I choose "good enough" over "never enough." That's my plan at least. And that, too, will have to be good enough.

One of the unexpected pleasures of my new mantra is the wealth of opportunities I have to practice it with my daughters. With my germ-phobic 13-year-old, things are clean enough: "that brownie was on the floor for 4 seconds . . . tops." With my 11-year-old who began rejecting all meat products several years ago, I bury the chicken broth can in the recycling bin, saying: "Just eat it, it's vegetarian enough."

For the first time in my life, I feel like I wouldn't be gypped if it all ended tomorrow. I ache at the thought that I would never hear my daughters' laughter again (though in my mind that will be my heaven), and I despair at the vision of my girls crying over life's joys and heartbreaks without me there to toast them or to comfort them. But now I don't fear being forgotten. I don't fear that I'll leave without having contributed in some small way. I don't fear what's around the bend. And I'm not beating myself up for what I haven't done or what I should be doing. Really. I'm just happy to float here for a while.

Jennifer Lear (42) is a lawyer who spent the last 13 years at home with her two daughters. She has recently returned to work full-time as a professor, teaching legal writing to first-year law students. Her husband hopes she'll return to the mega bucks of big firm practice someday (so he can retire), but instead she hopes to make her Broadway debut by 50.

Acknowledgments

Women in their 40s are in the maelstrom of balancing career, family, health, friends and the scarce time for themselves. That fact makes the all-volunteer nature of this book even more amazing to me. Every person involved in this book, from the writers to the editors, the designers and the web hosters, has donated their time to support this project and this cause. I was humbled and grateful. Whenever we needed something – content, cover design, even wine for the launch party – our request was met with an enthusiastic, "Sure, I would be happy to help!" virtually every time.

Thank you to my early contributors, Nancy Kho, Tina Goette, Liz Becker, Diane Perro, and Maria Hjelm, who made me confident that we really had a story to tell. Thank you to Jennifer Lear, for coming back into my life and bringing Lauren Bogart and Erin St. John Kelly into the fold. Thank you Kristin, for your enthusiasm to be part of the community and introducing me to Elaine Hamill. Thank you Kim and Liz, for initially helping to get the word out and introducing me to Esther Gulli. Thanks to Amy and Edie who provided a look at the work side of our lives. Thank you to LiteraryMama. com, BettyConfidential.com, Erinne O'Hara and WomenBloom. com for posting the Call for Submissions, bringing us submissions from women across the country, including Gabrielle Selz, Lori Stott, Mardi Link, Therese Gilardi, Stephanie Vanderslice, Regina Sewell,

Ona Gritz, Anita Drieseberg and Natalie Serber. Thanks to Susan, Vicki and Thea for responding to my email, and to Robin's sisters for allowing us to include her essay in this book.

We took an unconventional approach to editing, just as we've taken an unconventional approach to most aspects of this book. My Editorial Review Committee was important in providing an honest assessment of the essays, and helping to pick out a well-rounded collection. My heartfelt appreciation to Mira Ringler, Robin Brandt, Carrie Coltman, Ann Mamallo, Jami York, and especially to Debbie Bonzell who also connected me with Kym Miller and Ana Ammann. Samantha Pinney, not only are you a wonderful writer, you turned out excellent critiques as well. Cari, Kristin and Jennifer, you were great pinch hitters when I really needed you. Mary Pezzuto, you were a true partner in the editing process, spending hours and lending your editorial expertise to pull the comments together and asking the tough questions along the way.

Many thanks to Laura Batti, who was recuperating from radiation therapy when we met, and created an upbeat, unique design for the book, website and everything else; to Holly Stewart, our photographer, who jumped right into the fray; and to Maureen French, our stylist who took me under her wing in picking out looks and styles at Bloomingdales and Nordstroms. Thank you to the Ford Modeling Agency, who quickly responded to our request for help and sent two wonderful models, Jette and Nina, who donated their legs and their time. Thanks again to Nancy who showed that 40-something women can indeed still have great legs.

Thank you to Damon Wood and LMI Web Services who volunteered to get us on the web painlessly. Thanks to Jane Ahrens and Frank Henson who early on helped with a title, and to David Collins at WingSpan Press who led me through the unknown jungle of publishing.

My love and thanks to my family for putting up with my papers and computer spread across the dining room table for months, to Caleb and Ellie for getting over having Mom publish a book with the word *Sex* in the title, and to Seth for having the belief in me to first suggest that I develop this book when we walked out of the bookstore empty-handed on my 40th birthday a year ago.

Molly Tracy Rosen
Oakland, California

Individual Essay Copyright Information